'In this rich and prolific book Amir brings to our attention the many aspects of the relations between psychic processes and the principles of language. She casts a light on regions that are outside the reach of verbal expression or even clash with any effort at articulation. Her clinical innovations, anchored in her profound understanding of the mazes of psychic syntax, make a daring and original addition to the psychoanalytic canon.'

– **Prof. Aner Govrin,** *Doctoral Program in Psychoanalysis, Hermeneutics & Cultural Studies, Bar-Ilan University*

T0383439

# Psychoanalysis on the Verge of Language

This book examines the importance of language in psychoanalytic theory and practice, offering an understanding of how language can give a deeper insight into the psyche both in clinical practice and everyday life.

Bringing together psychoanalytic insights that hinge on the language of "difficult cases", this collection also includes contributions dedicated to meta-study of psychoanalytic writing. The first chapter shows how music includes tonal regions that deploy existing rules and syntax, alongside atonal ones dominated by caesuras, pauses and tensions. The second chapter discusses the malignant ambiguity of revealing and concealing typical of incestuous situations, pinpointing how the ambiguous language of incest "deceives by means of the truth". The third chapter brings in Virginia Woolf's character Orlando in order to illustrate two types of gender crossing. Distinctions defined by the linguist Roman Jakobson help in the fourth chapter to offer an integrative description of obsessive–compulsive phenomenon as an interaction between metaphoric and metonymic dimensions, as well as with a third, psychotic dimension. The fifth chapter focuses on what is called the "screen confessions" typical of the perpetrator's language. George Orwell's "newspeak" is used here to decipher the specific means by which the perpetrator turns his or her "inner witness" into a blind one. The final chapter uses Roland Barthes' concepts of "studium" and "punctum" to discuss the limits of psychoanalytic writing. As a whole, this book sets the psychoanalytic importance of language in a wider understanding of how language helps to shape and even create the internal as well as the external world.

Drawing on insights from psychoanalytic theory and practice, as well as from linguistics and cultural theory, this book will be invaluable for psychoanalysts, psychoanalytic psychotherapists and bibliotherapists, as well as anyone interested in how language forms our reality.

**Prof. Dana Amir** is a clinical psychologist, supervising and training analyst at the Israel psychoanalytic society, full professor and head of the interdisciplinary doctoral program in psychoanalysis at Haifa University, vice-dean for research, the Faculty of education at Haifa University, editor of *Maarag—the Israel Annual of Psychoanalysis* (the Hebrew University), poetess and literature researcher. Her previous nonfiction books are: *Cleft Tongue* (Karnac Books, 2014); *On the Lyricism of the mind* (Routledge, 2016); *Bearing Witness to the Witness* (Routledge, 2019).

# Psychoanalysis In A New Key Book Series

Donnel Stern
Series Editor

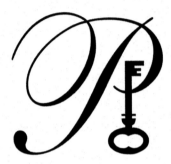

When music is played in a new key, the melody does not change, but the notes that make up the composition do: change in the context of continuity, a continuity that perseveres through change. Psychoanalysis in a New Key publishes books that share the aims psychoanalysts have always had, but that approach them differently. The books in the series are not expected to advance any particular theoretical agenda, although to this date most have been written by analysts from the Interpersonal and Relational orientations.

The most important contribution of a psychoanalytic book is the communication of something that nudges the reader's grasp of clinical theory and practice in an unexpected direction. Psychoanalysis in a New Key creates a deliberate focus on innovative and unsettling clinical thinking. Because that kind of thinking is encouraged by exploration of the sometimes surprising contributions to psychoanalysis of ideas and findings from other fields, Psychoanalysis in a New Key particularly encourages interdisciplinary studies. Books in the series have married psychoanalysis with dissociation, trauma theory, sociology and criminology. The series is open to the consideration of studies examining the relationship between psychoanalysis and any other field—for instance, biology, literary and art criticism, philosophy, systems theory, anthropology and political theory.

But innovation also takes place within the boundaries of psychoanalysis, and Psychoanalysis in a New Key therefore also presents work that reformulates thought and practice without leaving the precincts of the field. Books in the series focus, for example, on the significance of personal values in psychoanalytic practice, on the complex interrelationship between the analyst's clinical work and personal life, on the consequences for the clinical situation when patient and analyst are from different cultures, and on the need for psychoanalysts to accept the degree to which they knowingly satisfy their own wishes during treatment hours, often to the patient's detriment. A full list of all titles in this series is available at:

https://www.routledge.com/Psychoanalysis-in-a-New-Key-Book-Series/book-series/LEAPNKBS

# Psychoanalysis on the Verge of Language

## Clinical Cases on the Edge

Dana Amir

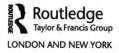
Routledge
Taylor & Francis Group

LONDON AND NEW YORK

First published 2022
by Routledge
2 Park Square, Milton Park, Abingdon, Oxon OX14 4RN

and by Routledge
605 Third Avenue, New York, NY 10158

*Routledge is an imprint of the Taylor & Francis Group, an informa business*

*British Library Cataloguing-in-Publication Data*
A catalogue record for this book is available from the British Library

*Library of Congress Cataloging-in-Publication Data*
Names: Amir, Dana, author.
Title: Psychoanalysis on the verge of language : clinical cases on the edge /Dana Amir.
Description: Milton Park, Abingdon, Oxon; New York, NY : Routledge, 2022. | Includes bibliographical references and index.
Identifiers: LCCN 2021012353 (print) | LCCN 2021012354 (ebook) | ISBN 9781032046488 (hardback) | ISBN 9781032023700 (paperback) | ISBN 9781003194071 (ebook)
Subjects: LCSH: Psycholinguistics. | Psychoanalysis.
Classification: LCC BF455 .A519 2022 (print) | LCC BF455 (ebook) | DDC 401/.9--dc23 LC record available at https://lccn.loc.gov/2021012353LC ebook record available at https://lccn.loc.gov/2021012354

ISBN: 978-1-032-04648-8 (hbk)
ISBN: 978-1-032-02370-0 (pbk)
ISBN: 978-1-003-19407-1 (ebk)

DOI: 10.4324/9781003194071

Typeset in Times New Roman
by MPS Limited, Dehradun

To Michael, Yuval and Michal

# Contents

# Acknowledgments

Every effort has been made to contact the copyright holders for their permission to reprint selections of this book. The publishers would be grateful to hear from any copyright holder who is not here acknowledged and will undertake to rectify any errors or omissions in future editions of this book.

This book was first published in Hebrew under the following title:
Amir, D. (2020). *Screen Confessions*. Tel-Aviv: Resling.
The Epilogue was published as part of a *Memoir* in Hebrew:
Amir, D. (2019). *Kaddish on Light and Darkness*. Tel-Aviv: Afik Books.
Chapter 1 was first published as the following paper and reprinted by permission:
Amir, D. (2017). Tonality and Atonality in the Psychic Space. *Journal of Poetry Therapy*, *30*(3), 166–174.
Chapter 2 was first published as the following paper and reprinted by permission:
Amir, D. (2019). The Malignant Ambiguity of Incestuous Language. *Contemporary Psychoanalysis*, *55*(3), 252–274.
Chapter 3 was first published as the following chapter and reprinted by permission:
Amir, D. (2018). The Two Sleeps of Orlando: Transsexuality as Caesura or Cut. In Oren Gozlan (Ed.). *Current Critical Debates in the Field of Transsexual Studies: In Transition*. London & New-York: Routledge, pp. 36–47.
Chapter 4 was first published as the following paper and reprinted by permission:

Amir, D. (2016). The Metaphoric, the Metonymic and the Psychotic Aspects of Obsessive-Sympomatology. *International Journal of Psychoanalysis*, *97*, 259–280.

Chapter 5 was first published as the following paper and reprinted by permission:

Amir, D. (2017). Screen Confessions: A Current Analysis of Nazi Perpetrators' 'Newspeak'. *Psychoanalysis, Culture & Society*, *23*(1), 97–114.

The Epilogue was first published as the following paper and reprinted by permission:

Amir, D. (2018). 'Punctum' and 'Studium' in Psychoanalytic Writing: Reading Case Studies Through Roland Barthes. *Psychoanalytic Review*, *105*(1), 51–65.

# Foreword

*Aner Govrin*

Dana Amir's psychoanalytic thinking has been with us for nearly two decades, gaining itself a faithful readership in the psychoanalytic community in Israel as well as abroad. The profound significance of her work, her place in the psychoanalytic thinking of her times, her specific take on object relations theory, and her unique poetic and linguistic perspective invite due attention.

Dana Amir's psychoanalytic thinking combines a constant search for psychic truth with the attempt to create an esthetic-linguistic vehicle capable of capturing that truth. I would like to call her genre "scientific-poetic". Scientific, because it has been psychoanalysis' project, from the start, to describe the facts or foundations of the psyche. Though it operates on complex principles and rules, whether implicit or explicit, they are, as such, stable and amenable to conceptualization. These principles—including the unconscious, the etiology of hysteria and the neuroses, intra-psychic dynamics, object relations, defense mechanisms, transference, projective identification and so on—can be described as if they actually had an existence in external reality, namely as though they were natural phenomena. The conditions from which they evolve, their fundamentally rule-bound nature, and the mental processes they set into motion can all be described. Efforts at such a description, however, come hardly ever in dry scientific language: they deploy poetic tools. Here words do not simply carry contents: the way in which they are put together and the resulting emotional resonance render the subject matter esthetically. The truth value of psychoanalytic discoveries therefore depends on the poetic skill and expressiveness of the one who conveys them.

We can place psychoanalytic authors on a sequence stretching between a scientific style that faithfully reproduces an orthodox, correct and highly polished psychoanalytic jargon, and poetic language relying on the musical characteristics of the words, on suggestive imagery, surprising metaphors, and more than anything, as in the case of Amir's writing, a musical sensibility that turns every reading into a musical performance in its own right.

The side of scientific jargon is represented by authors like Klein, Kernberg, Mahler and Masterson, while Winnicott, Eigen, Philips and Milner can be seen on the other, poetic side of psychoanalytic writing style. Regardless of where any given author is located on this continuum, their text will always display a certain blend between the genres. Each in her or his own way seeks to describe the "facts" of the psyche while also and at the same time allowing the reader to concretely try and sample psychic materials.

It is here, in regard to these qualities, that Amir's voice is extraordinary. A former musician and currently a renowned poet, Dana Amir is more than anything an incomparably subtle and accomplished reader of literature and an expert on music. She approaches literature, including poetry, as a real site where we experience the psyche's hidden as well as manifest qualities, thus producing a unique additional layer of understanding to clinical situations and phenomena. She constructs a coherent approach which, by organizing psychic materials in linguistic terms, helps us connect and illustrate both the normative and the eccentric phenomena we encounter in the clinic. In this she continues an important tradition initiated by authors like Julia Kristeva, Jacques Lacan and Luce Irigaray.

From this point of entry Dana Amir challenges psychoanalytic thinking, which tended to refer to the clinical situation: she develops and expands an additional resource which complements the description of inner reality. She describes deep structures and poetic mechanisms which also reflect the principles, facts and implicit rules driving the psyche. Amir's perspective adds a unique interdisciplinary angle to psychoanalysis' conceptual reservoir. Since literary prose and poetry, too, speak in the name of what is concealed, and since like psychoanalysis, they do not bring a rational interpretation to reality, these texts too may lay bare psychic rules and principles. Amir shows us how this yields insights on a par with those we derive from our clinical work.

Her books and articles, therefore, by offering us a linguistic toolbox, show the reader roads hitherto not taken. Amir points out how literary-linguistic modes of representation can hone our description and understanding of both psychic processes and their healing. Tonal and atonal musical structures, harmony and disharmony, levels of metaphoricity—emerge as formative of the psyche's deep processes. Amir's unique introduction of musical and linguistic discursivities takes the psychoanalytic reader into new territories.

The present collection of articles brings together deep psychoanalytic insights that all hinge on the language of what we call "difficult cases", for example: the three dimensions of the obsessional phenomenon; the malignant ambiguity of incestuous language; the characteristics of the victimizer's language and the interrelations between actual and phantasmatic gender. At the same time, this collection includes contributions dedicated to a kind of meta-study of psychoanalytic writing as such. Amir navigates between the linguistic and musical coordinates which she evolves as a confident and experienced clinician. In the first chapter, she shows how music includes tonal regions that deploy existing rules and syntax, alongside atonal ones dominated by caesuras, pauses and tensions; the latter have an effect of constant motion and an ongoing search. These musical coordinates help Amir to describe a psychic reality given to a constant tension, too, between saturated, familiar conditions and unsaturated ones that carry a potential for risk but also for change. In this respect, Amir points out regions of psychic modulation, marked by transposition, as opposed to regions of psychic transformation, characterized by true change. In the second chapter, Amir discusses the malignant ambiguity of revealing and concealing typical of incestuous situations. She makes an attempt unprecedented in the professional literature to pinpoint how the ambiguous language of incest "deceives by means of the truth", or disguises itself as if it facilitated connection while in fact attacking any possibility to connect. In her third chapter, Amir brings in Virginia Woolf's character Orlando to illustrate two types of gender crossing: one exemplifies a type of crossing she identifies as "caesura", which transforms what she calls "gender excess", as opposed to a type of crossing she identifies as "cut", which itself is an acting out, rather than a transformation, of this gender excess. Distinctions defined by the linguist Roman Jakobson help Amir in her fourth chapter to offer an integrative description of obsessive–compulsive disorder as an interaction between metaphoric and metonymic aspects, as well as with a third, psychotic aspect which she adds herself. In this disorder, these three aspects combine in various, specific ways. Amir shows how clinical work with this disorder can gain from mapping out the particular interaction between them, allowing in that way an appropriate interpretive mode. In the fifth chapter, Amir deciphers what she calls the syntax of the perpetrator's language. Here she puts forward George Orwell's newspeak, a notion he used to suggest how history—factual and affective—gets rewritten. She also refers to Hannah Arendt's expression of "the banality of evil" in order to show how perpetrators in their "screen confessions" dodge the problematic nature of their acts. "By dismantling the language in which they think their actions, perpetrators exclude not only the victims from the story but themselves as well. As long as the perpetrator remains outside the story, her or his testimonial text constitutes an "empty event" or an "event without witness"—an event from which the perpetrator, allegedly the most reliable witness of her or his own actions, is absent" (ibid). In the sixth and final chapter, Amir uses Roland Barthes' concepts of *Studium* and *Punctum* to discuss the limits of psychoanalytic writing as such. Barthes' notions here serve as touchstones for the relations between the psychoanalytic-cultural context which the clinical vignette is recruited to confirm (studium) and those cases where the clinical vignette comes to question and puncture the fabric of that context (punctum) in order to free up a new space for thought. Here Amir elaborates a typical failure of psychoanalytic writing: while tending to rely on linearity and coherence it loses the "puncturing" potential of the psychoanalytic vignette, its capacity to smuggle a "wild element" into the well-structured scene—one that refuses to align with the accepted cultural syntax rules.

In this rich and prolific book Amir brings to our attention the many aspects of the relations between psychic processes and the principles of language. She casts a light on regions that are outside the reach of verbal expression or even clash with any effort at articulation. Her clinical innovations, anchored in her profound understanding of the mazes of psychic syntax, make a daring and original addition to the psychoanalytic canon.

# Prologue: The body is all ears

During my childhood vacations, my father used to take us to the forests so we could listen to the nature with our eyes closed. Each of us was told to catch a sound and listen to it in isolation from all the other sounds. The twittering of one bird among the rest, the sound made by the branches of a shrub brushing against each other, the rustle of dry leaves on the ground.

Why did we shut our eyes? Because hearing and seeing get in each other's way. Vision tends to take over the perceptual domain, concealing, or perhaps camouflaging, what the other senses might have picked up from the general jumble of stimuli. Hearing, by contrast, is tricky. It may be hard to tell whether a sound originates inside or out. When, in an auditorium full of people, someone raises his hand—there is no room for mistakes. But when someone speaks up without indicating where they are located, their voice sometimes appears to come from nowhere near where they actually are. Sounds converse with each other. They pour into one another.

Closing our eyes we allow hearing to be the soloist in the orchestra of our senses. When an environment is perceived solely, or mainly, through hearing, its various frequencies signal not just the provenance of the sound but also our own location in space. Isolating the twittering of one bird is not the same as locating the bird. It means that we use its returning chirps to place ourselves in relation to it.

Lying on the dry soil, I close my eyes. The first sound I notice is my sister's and brothers' breathing, as they lie next to me. My sister giggles. My middle brother breathes so quietly his breath almost blends with the wind. The little one, however, is panting heavily, his nose seemingly blocked. Afraid to be lost he tries to situate himself in the space through the sound of his own breathing. The wind makes the pine branches above us tremble. Thin pine needles fall onto my face. I try to remove them without using my fingers, by pursing my lips only. Their smell is strong, intoxicating.

The sound of a pine cone falling on the ground. The tiny sound of a beetle's feet in the grass. Slowly, the clusters of sound begin to come apart. The sound of one beetle's feet separates from that of another's. The pine cone produces a different sound depending on whether it falls on its face or on its side. Each of these sounds resonates differently in the various parts of my body. The sound of the pine cone transforms my spine into an audio channel, while the sound of the beetle's feet tickles the tip of my nose. The body is all ears.

I have always paid attention to the way sounds are produced by the speaking mouth. For some people speech is a huge effort. Words leave their mouths tensely, tied on both sides, and that's how they reach the hearer too: encrusted, turned inward. For others, speech is a kind of concealment. One word is immediately joined to the next, and the connection between them is a connection by the grace of dis-traction—nothing more: they deflect the hearer's ear from what is said to speaking itself. Finally, there are those who cast their words with a skillful hand like exact arrows. This ejection requires a certain delay in the production of the voice itself, a voice whose strings must be impeccably tuned. When words are produced that way, they create, no matter their content, a presentation of total necessity.

The body is an amplifier that conveys sounds. When, as young children, we'd put an ear to one of our parents' bellies, a whole orch-estra of sounds would make itself heard. Our own bellies, too, were vocal. When we slept together on the beach, during summer vacations, these dull rumblings from the small bellies near me, would signal a wakeful presence in the sleeping tent. These sounds had a calming effect, similar to that of the waves coming and going on the beach. Cyclicity itself, one in which the digestive system features as an extension of the solar system, seat of the motions of ebb and flow, seat of the seasons, inspired me with a kind of calm.

Music was part of this cyclicity. I always listened to sounds from both sides. There was the absolute sound, which approached me together with its proper name. And there was the relative sound, which resided to the back of the absolute sound and which could, suddenly, turn into a screech, a murmur, a sigh. That's why I always preferred the chromatic scale. The chromatic structure captured something of the hidden side of sounds. Making music was creating an equation with many variables while also refusing a solution. This refusal, for me, was music's very condition of existence—exactly because music, essentially, invites absolute devotion.

For many years, I played only by ear. The printed notes seemed to me like a barrier, barbed wire, keeping me away from music itself. Sounds passed from my ears to my fingers and back again, without any involvement of my eyes. And because I played with closed eyes my encounters with sounds were, as it were, formal: at the tips of my fingers they came to shape a ball, a jug, or a flower. They poured into each other, pushed against each other. My encounter with them was not that of a seeing person, who extracts meaning from revealed outlines—but that of a listener, who first extracts meaning, and only then draws its outlines in her imagination.

Music, for me, was the thing itself. I don't mean the art of music, but the art of life which music, perhaps, renders most powerfully: a criterion of listening that emerges in contrast with the perception of reality.

Listening to music constitutes a space between eye and ear that challenges the basic rules. Here what's left behind and won't return lies enfolded. Perhaps because in it, as the forests of my childhood have taught me, the human point of departure is most plainly borne out: we are all ears.

# Chapter 1

# Tonality and atonality in the psychic space

The term tonality, or tonal harmony, covers most of the music composed in Europe from the mid-17th century until the end of the 19th, as well as the major part of popular western music from the 20th century onwards. Simply put, tonal music is harmonious music, following the laws of harmony and obeying the expectations of the western ear (Xenakis, 1992; Zimmerman, 2002). Atonality,[1] by contrast, denotes music written anytime from the early 20th century, which does not refer to a tonal center. This music does not conform to the typical tonal hierarchy of western classical music, and—naturally—does not meet the expectations of the western ear: it is not harmonious, its movements are not predictable, and it operates outside the familiar musical rules and scales.

Tonality and atonality may be rephrased as "syntax" and "anti-syntax". If tonality is a condition in which the musical text obeys the known syntactic rules and hence, alongside the specific emotional range it institutes, also inspires a sense of familiarity and orientation—atonality challenges the familiar rules, creating an alien, uncanny environment in which the listener's ear finds it hard to orient itself. If tonality is grounded in a stable scale whose sounds are arranged in a clear order and which marks the starting point of the musical work to which it returns—then atonality occurs when the "tonal center" is absent. This absence generates the use of ambiguous chords, unusual harmonic, melodic, and rhythmic inflections, lacking a point of departure and return. If tonality represents the homely, then atonality points to the un-homely, Freud's (1919) *das Unheimliche*. It is generally assumed that tonality is a natural feature of the human brain and that the mind unintentionally searches for tonal

DOI: 10.4324/9781003194071-1

centers while listening to music. This is why we feel uncomfortable when we encounter atonal music, which the "tonal ear" experiences as a jarring noise or disturbance.

Poetry (or the poetic zones of literature in general) is a unique expression of the integration of tonal and atonal linguistic zones. On the one hand—it speaks through words, which are basically "tonal" units (intelligible, common); on the other hand, it uses these tonal units in such an original and unpredictable way that the resulting text is characterized by a marked atonal tendency of different intensities and kinds: one which transgresses its own limits and thus plays out of its own scale. The poetic zones of psychoanalysis and psychotherapy are in that sense therapeutic forces which pull toward atonal psychic areas, enabling the ongoing integration of the homely and un-homely, the syntax and the anti-syntax of the psychic space.

This chapter looks at the psyche's inclination toward tonal centers, and at the way in which mental atonality subverts experiences of centeredness while simultaneously producing unsaturated spaces which are no less vital to it than the tonal ones. The relation between tonal and atonal aspects in the psychic space determines the relations between movement and stasis. In its best, tonality pulls toward a sense of centeredness, while in its worst it drags toward fixation. Extreme cases of atonality, on the other hand, may issue in a disintegration of continuity. But in its favorable manifestations atonality vitally undermines saturated hierarchies, thereby enriching the psychic texture.

In the psychic space, like in music, atonal regions hold contradictions, inherent tensions and ambivalence, which do not pull toward an immediate and intelligible solution. While both holding and producing tension, these regions also give rise to a movement of constant searching. Where there is an excess of such areas with no ability to generate a tonal solution, an experience of fragmentation may emerge, resulting from the lack of a psychic center. A paucity, or absence, of these regions, on the other hand, may result in fixation in the shape of saturated thinking and a tendency toward saturated solutions.

In an unpublished paper entitled "Catastrophic Change" (1967)—later reprinted as "Container and Contained Transformed" (1970)—Bion describes the interaction between what he defines as "the Establishment" (representing the stable, sometimes rigid force that resists change) and "the messianic idea" (which represents the force of innovation and change), arguing that the aspect of the personality which always stays stable and fixed is actually the only force that can contain new perceptions of the self and of the world:

> The individual always displays some aspect of his personality that is stable and constant even though it may sometimes be very difficult to detect in the welter of evidence for instability; it may appear only in the regularity with which the patient attends his sessions. In this stability will be found the counterpart of what [..] I have called the Establishment. It will be maintained with great tenacity as the only force likely to contain the counterpart of the messianic idea. Reciprocally, the messianic idea is the only force likely to withstand the pressures of the counterpart of the Establishment in the individual. (1970, p. 121)

Bion further points at three possible types of interaction between the establishment and the messianic idea which he calles "symbiotic", "commensal" and "parasitic":

> I shall not trouble with the commensal relationship: the two sides coexist and the existence of each can be seen to be harmless to the other. In the symbiotic relationship there is a confrontation and the result is growth producing though that growth may not be discerned without some difficulty. In the parasitic relationship, the product of the association is something that destroys both parties to the association. (Ibid, p. 78)

Assuming that the influence of the atonal regions on the tonal ones is similar to the influence of the messianic idea on the establishment, the relations between tonal and atonal psychic areas may be rephrased, using Bion's terminology, as follows: Where a parasitical interaction occurs between the tonal and atonal psychic zones—destructive relations may arise between atonal tension and the yearning for a harmonious solution. When the subjective experience is that the tonal tendency blocks any transcendence of it—or alternatively, that such a transcendence puts paid to the possibility of a harmonious solution—then tonality and atonality become mutually exclusive. Commensal relationship, on the other hand, make possible the existence, side by side, of tonal and atonal psychic zones—even though a connection or link between them does not always exist. Here, harmonious regions assume an insular shape and so do atonal regions. Neither nourishing nor clashing with one another, they maintain a kind of status quo which while not culminating in conflict does not enable significant new development either. It is only in the symbiotic relationship that a struggle occurs which allows tonal areas to contain the threatening atonal areas in a way that eventually holds a possibility for growth and change. Atonality forms the greatest danger to tonality, yet constitutes the only force that can bring about a new tonality and in that sense promote the tonal center exactly by its transcendence.

Tonality and atonality do not only characterize psychic regions but may also characterize forms of internalization of the primary object. Could it be that some psyches are born with an a priori atonal tendency while others are characterized by an a priori fundamental and stable tonal center? What are the implications of such inborn tendencies for the relations with the primary object?

One might consider the interaction within the primary dyad as a reflection of a certain relation between the tonal and atonal aspects of both the primary object and the infant. Objects whose atonal dimension dominates tend to engender an experience of tension and restlessness, a lack of center and harmonious stability. Such a primary object is bound to instill an inherent ambivalence and tension in the primary dyad which may in turn affect the infantile psyche. But there are the a priori characteristics of the infant as well: Some infants are born with an inherent atonality, that is, with a weaker and less stable ability to internalize the object's tonality, while other infants whose natural tonality is strong enough are much more capable to endure atonal deviations, both in the object and in themselves. An essentially "tonal" infant will obviously be better able to tolerate atonal regions in the primary dyad as well as in him or herself. Hence this infant will be less distraught, than an "atonal" infant who depends much more on the dominant tonality of the primary object. A tonal infant will also gain more from contact with atonal regions, while an atonal infant will be very much in need of the tonality of the other. These relations, clearly, are not static. They change throughout the years of development. At some points, or during some phases, the need for tonality takes precedence and becomes critical, while in other areas and at other times there appears to be more space for atonality. The ability to demarcate or posit a center is necessary to any ability to deviate from it. It may happen though that tonal centrality comes to predominate, turning one's entire discourse into something that no longer tolerates new movement. When tonal centrality takes over the therapeutic discourse, for instance, there is a danger that both analytic interpretation and analytic thinking may collapse, time and again, into the same exhausted "tonality". Not only the specific analytic discourse may crash under its own tonal centrality—the broader meta-analytic discourse, too, can founder under its own familiar coordinates.

Such a collapse can be witnessed in the mechanical repetition of tonal centers or familiar theoretical scales, depending on the theoretical-tonal environment from which one has evolved: the Freudian Oedipal triangle (Freud, 1924), Kleinian positions (Klein, 1952), Winnicottian potential space (Winnicott, 1971), Kohutian primary deficit (Kohut, 1971), and so on—all serve as coordinates, productively forming the outlines of our thinking but also constraining it.

In contrast with this collapse into the known tonal coordinates, atonal freedom may be thought of as taking us away from the familiar scales, forcing us to diverge from the equations we usually form. The psychic counterpoint, as well as the analytic one, are determined by the relation between tonality and atonality, which simultaneously preserve outlines and their inbuilt tension, the pull toward linking as well as the inherent threat to any existing link.

Atonality is human idiosyncrasy. This idiosyncrasy which tends to be considered negatively in tonal psychoanalytic tradition as regions of nonthinking or as an expression of lack of psychic center—is also a critical source of power. This is the power to escape not only the ready-made categories which the world presents us but also the categories in which we, subtly and repeatedly, ensnare ourselves. Idiosyncratic areas that resist explanation are a proof of the existence of an unstoppable life force—one that breaks its way right across all beaten tracks to enable the ex-territory required for any territory to exist. In music, in psychoanalysis, in philosophy—the most exciting zones are those where an unsaturated atonal element subverts a saturated tonal one. I am not thinking of where such a movement results in a new "saturated solution"—but of those situations in which it remains an unsaturated element at the very center of the saturated space of thinking, a source of discomfort within the serene, a sound whose discordance does not shatter the general experience yet deposits a permanently ambivalent dimension.

One of the most beautiful examples of this type of idiosyncrasy can be observed in the poetic language of Clarice Lispector, an excellent representative of the deviation from conventions and central tonality. Her writing generates a magnetic field whose strength inheres in the uncanniness it creates, always refusing to be subsumed, resolved, or to settle down in the linearity of worn-out formulas.

At the opening of her story "The Foreign Legion" (1984) a family is seated around the table on which there is a chick they were given. A mother, father, and four sons are looking at the helpless chick, as they try in vain to find the "right" attitude in the face of its frightened squeaks:

> There we were, and no one was worthy of appearing before a chick; with every chirp it drove us away. With each chirp, it reduced us to helplessness. The constancy of its terror accused us of a thoughtless merriment which by now was no longer merriment, but annoyance. The chick's moment had passed, and with ever greater urgency it banished us while keeping us imprisoned.
>
> (Lispector, 1992, p. 88)

Lispector shines a light on a scene, which could have easily been tonal: the chick's tenderness and helplessness calling forth a corresponding tenderness, compassion and wish to cradle it in those seated around the table. She, however, offers us this scene from its atonal, alien, uncanny perspective. From being a spot of light, the chick transforms into a sinister signifier: from something that enables and releases the tenderness of the family members around the table it turns to something that terrorizes them with its helplessness, its dread chasing them away and holding them spellbound at the same time:

> As for the chick, it was chirping. Standing on the polished table, it dared not make a move as it chirped from within. I never knew that so much terror could exist inside a creature that was made

only of feathers. Feathers covering what? Half a dozen fragile little bones which had been loosely put together for what reason? To chirp terror. [...] It was impossible to give the chick those words of reassurance which would allay its fears and bring consolation to that creature which was terrified just to have been born. How could one promise it protection? A father and a mother, we knew just how brief the chick's life would be. The chick also knew, in the way that living creatures know; through profound fear. (pp. 88–89)

And thus, Lispector marks fear as bringing us close to our deepest knowledge of ourselves rather than removing us from it. This is how we know. Not through the moments when we love, that is, when we are firmly placed at the umbilicus of our inner space, but when we are cast outside ourselves, finding ourselves in an alien scene which may unfold in the most familiar place, the home, a scene in which we are cast in roles that are foreign to anything we ever thought—or wanted to think—of ourselves. Lispector's solution never strays into a familiar tonality. She insists on singing off the formal scale, to pave a path that strays away. This straying, however, does not necessarily lead to an abyss:

The younger boy could stand it no longer:
Do you want to be its mummy?
Startled, I answered yes. I was the messenger assigned to that creature which did not understand the only language I knew: I was loving without being loved. My mission was precarious and the eyes of four children waited with the intransigence of hope for my first gesture of effective love. I recoiled a little, smiling and solitary. [...] I tried to isolate myself from the challenge of those five males, so that I, too, might expect love from myself and remember what love is like. I opened my mouth, I was about to tell them the truth: exactly how, I cannot say.
But if a woman were to appear to me in the night holding a child in her lap. And if she were to say: Take care of my child. I would reply: How can I? She would repeat: Take care of my child. I would reply: I cannot. She would insist: Take care of my child. Then—then, because I do not know how to do anything and because I cannot remember

anything and because it is night—then I would stretch out my hand and save a child. Because it is night, because I am alone in another person's night, because this silence is much too great for me, because I have two hands in order to sacrifice the better of the two, and because I have no choice.

So I stretched out my hand and held the chick. (pp. 89–90)

Lispector's atonal solution manages to gain hold from an unusual direction. Here hold does not flow from responsibility, a sense of obligation or from love or an omnipotent fantasy of redemption. The hand that holds the chick is helpless exactly like it, and it is only due to this helplessness, which does not disguise itself as power, knowledge or willful decision, that it can claim this hold. In this grip, power derives from the absence of power: "...because I am alone in another person's night", namely, because I was willing to be a guest in the other person's helplessness, or in the other person's ignorance, or rather—because I could not but diverge from myself into this strange "night" of the stranger in front of me, because of this, and only because of this, could I hold out my hand.

Lispector's atonality does not drop the narrator into the abyss but rather enables her to cross it. This abyss extends not merely between herself and the chick, between herself and her children, or between herself and the woman who appears in the middle of the night, demanding that she takes care of her child. It is the abyss within herself that she must cross here, the one preceding the abyss between herself and any other. Lispector's uniqueness inheres exactly in this lucid recognition of the chasm stretching between us and what is outside ourselves, and no less poignantly between us and what we experience as ours. Every hand offered, every word, every step—are a hand, a word, a step *as against* this abyss from within which Lispector's language speaks. This is why she doesn't slip into the usual formulas, those which can explain the narrator's reluctance to reach for either chick or the woman's child, by reference, for instance, to childhood events. Instead she captures the moment of helplessness and observes it outside any continuity, as an insulated existential unit which in its very exterritoriality enfolds the umbilicus of existence, and thus illuminates it.

Literature comes into its own exactly at these points, where it departs from the seductions of any ready-made formula. Psychoanalysis, similarly, comes to life at such a juncture. For it is sometimes exactly where one departs from the ability to describe oneself by means of routine formulations—moving into a domain that resists reduction to any of the conventional modes of explanation—that one achieves one's fullness of being.

I would like to conclude with some thoughts about atonality and modulation, their interrelations and their difference: *musical modulation* refers to the transition from one tonality to another, or from one musical key to another (Jones, 1994). Often, in modulation the motif manifested in the previous key—that is, in the previous tonal environment—is now played in a different key, namely, recreated in a new tonal environment. Even if there is no other change than this, the shift from one key to another, or from one tonal environment to another, produces a sense of freshness, renewal, a different affective climate. More stable musical parts are marked by less modulations while more "tense" ones usually feature more modulations in terms of both quantity and frequency.

What, then, is modulation in the context of the psychic space?

Often, in analysis as in everyday life—we create a modulation, which we experience as a transcendence, while what's really happening is that the tonal center, rather than disappearing altogether, shifts from one register to another. In other words, while departing from the original tonal center, modulation is not a departure from tonality as such. In this sense, with modulation we create the familiar tonality in a new environment (a new language, a new place, a new relationship). Even though the shift from one tonality to another always results in a certain tension, interest and an at least temporary sense of emotional uplift, it does not constitute a transcendence of the inner tonality but rather a transposition of it from one region to another.

A full deviation from the tonal center, in contrast, does not issue in the search for a new center but leads into a state in which the center as such is relinquished. This enables dwelling in a state of no-center while listening to the new possibilities this generates. This comes at the expense of familiarity and satisfaction; it will probably cause a sense of alienation, not just from the external world but also from one's inner experience of continuity. The experience could be likened to the unexpected encounter with our reflection in a mirror: it takes a moment until we realize that what we see is our own image; this moment allows us to observe ourselves from a distance both esthetic and affective, with a gaze free of desire and memory. It is an atonal moment in which we deviate absolutely, albeit for a split second, from the categories that constitute our self-perception. Yet, exactly because of its alien nature, this moment also gives rise to an un-paralleled intimate encounter with ourselves.

Musicologists have long tried to define the "procedures" from which atonal music emerges, identifying four of them in Schoenberg's work. Rather than rules, these procedures constitute "negative rules" in the sense that they focus on the don'ts rather than do's. In other words, atonal music does not constitute a structured new genre but is rather a negative engagement with the existing one.

This shines an especially interesting light on both the analytic context and reality outside the consulting room: The atonal regions of the psychic space do not introduce a new order (the ones that introduce a new order are in fact zones of modulation rather than zones of atonal transformation)—but quite the contrary: they subvert regularity as such, which is why, as mentioned, they are defined rather as the negation of what preceded them. But rather than a destructive negation, this is a creative deconstruction, undertaking the task of the disappropriation of the a hegemonicy and fixation of old formulas. Atonal psychic movement is not driven by the substitution of one genre by another, but by divergence from the generic as such. This may result in the most immediate contact with things in their very alienness, and hence in their very truthfulness.

In a chapter dedicated to the nature of esthetic judgment, the psy-choanalyst Donald Meltzer and the literary scholar Meg Harris-Williams suggest that in the encounter between self and object two modes of contact come into play: *carving* and *enveloping* (Meltzer and Harris-Williams, 1988, pp. 186–187; see also Amir, 2016). When the human mind encounters a new object it performs two actions, either in succession or simultaneously. On the one hand it "envelops" the new object in a familiar context, and on the other it encounters the object as absolutely and wholly alien. Taking Meltzer and Harris's notions one step further—it isn't merely the object that at this moment of encounter is experienced as familiar or alien but also the mind which experiences itself, through this object, in terms of familiarity or alienness. As it envelops the object in a familiar context the psyche reconfirms its own familiarity; when, however, it confronts the object in its alienness the encounter is with the alien aspect of itself.

This is why in the therapeutic text, it is the moment when language breaks down that is the most crucial. Not the moment in which one language replaces another, but the one in which there is a departure from language itself.

A while ago I was asked to comment on a vignette in which a patient suddenly kneeled in front of his analyst at the end of an analytic session. Within tonal psychoanalytic thinking, this moment might be seen to reflect a host of familiar coordinates: one might see it as a moment of seduction (the classic marriage proposal), a moment of infantile regression or a moment of psychic collapse.

But in the present context I would like to consider this moment as "atonal" in the sense that what it represents—before any meaning or content—is the disintegration of the form preceding it. A brave or desperate attempt to escape the central tonality of understanding and interpretation, the rituals of meeting and leaving, into a region that is unstructured by familiar categories and therefore demands new thinking: a shake-up of the stable tonal center of both analyst and analysis, calling into being, by means of this subversion, an area of intimate strangeness that requires no words.

## Note

1 The term atonality was coined by Joseph Marx in 1907.

## References

Amir, D. (2016). *On the Lyricism of the Mind: Psychoanalysis and Literature.* London: Routledge.

Bion, W. R. (1967). Catastrophic Change. Unpublished paper.

Bion, W. R. (1970). *Attention and Interpretation.* London: Tavistock [Reprinted London: Karnac Books, 1984.]

Freud, S. (1919). The 'Uncanny'. *The Standard Edition of the Complete Psychological Works of Sigmund Freud, Volume XVII (1917–1919): An Infantile Neurosis and Other Works.* London: The Hogarth Press, pp. 217–256.

Freud, S. (1924). *The Dissolution of the Oedipus Complex. The Standard Edition of the Complete Psychological Works of Sigmund Freud, Volume*

*XIX (1923–1925): The Ego and the Id and Other Works.* London: The Hogarth Press, pp. 171–180.

Jones, George T. (1994). *HarperCollins College Outline Music Theory.* New York: HarperCollins, p. 217.

Klein, M. (1952). Some Theoretical Conclusions Regarding the Emotional Life of the Infant. In *Developments in Psycho-analysis with Heimann, Isaacs and Rivière.* London: Hogarth.

Kohut, H. (1971). *The Analysis of the Self.* New York: International Universities Press.

Lispector, C. (1992). *The Foreign Legion* (trans., Giovanni Pontiero). New York: New Directions.

Matte Blanco, I. (1975). *The Unconscious as Infinite Sets. An Essay in Bi-logic.* London: Duckworth.

Meltzer, D., & Harris-Williams, M. (1988). Holding the Dream. In *The Apprehension of Beauty.* Scotland: Clunie Press, pp. 178–199.

Winnicott, D. W. (1971). *Playing and Reality.* New York: Basic Books.

Xenakis, Iannis. (1992; 1971). *Formalized Music: Thought and Mathematics in Composition.* Bloomington and London: Indiana University Press. Harmonologia Series No. 6. Stuyvesant, NY: Pendragon Press.

Zimmerman, Daniel J. (2002). *Families without Clusters in the Early Works of Sergei Prokofiev.* Unpublished PhD dissertation. Chicago: University of Chicago.

# Chapter 2

# The malignant ambiguity of incestuous language

The language of incest is ambiguous. The first to discuss this ambiguity was Ferenczi (1949), who showed how in the scene of the "confusion of tongues" the adult, under the cover of loving playfulness, uses the child to satisfy his desires, shifting from the language of tenderness to the language of passion. As a result, the child internalizes the aggressor, who transforms into an internal mental reality. Identification with the aggressor means that not only does the child do what he is expected to do but he also feels what he is expected to feel—whether this consists of identification with what the aggressor wants the child to feel, or with what he, the aggressor himself, feels. Thus, the child may experience the aggressor's desire as his own, and thereby participate in the pleasure and guilt the aggressor derives from abusing him or her.

In this present chapter, I discuss yet another ambiguity typical of incestuous language: the ambiguity of revealing and concealing. Here, ambiguity is generated by a language that pretends to produce meaning and enable links, but in fact constitutes a violent attack on linking (Bion, 1959). This is a language that deceives by using truth: under the cover of revealing truth it serves to screen that truth. This constitutes, in Laplanche's terms, an attack on the subject's function of translation.

According to Laplanche, a "fundamental anthropological situation" characterizes the human infant who comes into the world in a state of helplessness, a state which, under normal circumstances, is adequately made up for by the mother or her equivalent. Unless the situation is catastrophic, the infant easily understands and integrates parental

DOI: 10.4324/9781003194071-2

messages relating to basic needs. However, there is always a surplus, an excess, a "noise" in the communication stemming from the fundamental asymmetry between the two partners, which is not understood and integrated harmoniously. This communicational noise is the mystifying, repressed presence of the adult's sexuality, which is bound to contaminate the channels of communication, conveying a meaning that is enigmatic for both child and parent. This failure of translation is inevitable and denotes a process of repression. The unconscious is made up of the inassimilable remnants, the residues of the failed translations of the other's messages. Laplanche refers to such a process, which he calls *implantation*, as general seduction, the inevitable result of the adult-infant interaction, given the asymmetry between their respective psychic structures (Laplanche, 1989; Scarfone, 2013). When it comes to the pathogenic aspects of seduction, Laplanche refers to *intromission* as opposed to *implantation*: implantation is a neurotic process which allows the individual to engage actively, at once translating and repressing. Intromission, on the other hand, is its violent variant which puts an element resistant to all metabolization into the subject's interior (1998, p. 136). By depositing elements that are resistant to metabolization and thus fundamentally resistant to translation, intromission cripples the apparatus of translation itself, generating enclaves which strain the subject's psychic development (Scarfone, 2013).

Incest can be understood, in light of Laplanche's theory, as an extremely traumatic case of intromission. The incestuous seduction scene may be said to involve an attack that has fatal consequences not only for the child's ability to translate the specific messages of the specific other, but rather for his or her ability to perform the function of translation in general, that is, to create meaning and respond creatively to the enigmatic texture of human language. Instead, a fabric emerges that defends against any manifestation of enigmatic qualities, both in the other and in the self.

I would like to propose that the attack the incestuous scene causes involves not only the insertion of an element that resists translation—as Laplanche put it—but also the creation of a malignant ambiguity that pretends to encourage the function of translation while in fact paralyzing it. This malignant ambiguity contaminates any encounter with obscurity or perplexity that require translation and interpretation, thereby transforming interpretable elements into various types of threat which the psyche will attempt to repel or undo. Since in this ambiguous scene the child's mind is robbed of the ability to extricate meaning, the child becomes vulnerable to all kinds of penetration which he or she cannot moderate by means of thinking. In fact, thinking itself becomes a malignantly invaded and invasive region. Thinking demands an interaction between a thought and a thinker (Bion, 1959, 1962a, 1962b, 1970), i.e. an act of impregnation (as a consequence of which the current thought reverts into a preconception, i.e., into an open container seeking to contain yet another thought), and so depends on the capacity of elements of the personality to penetrate and be penetrated. In the case of incest, this necessary combination of active penetration and passive penetrability turns thinking itself into a threatened and threatening region. This involves an unconscious prohibition not on any specific thought, but on thinking as such, that is, on any interaction between container and contained. As a defense against this interaction a two-dimensional mental organization emerges.

Meltzer's main claim concerning two-dimensionality (1975) is that it is a type of mental functioning in which internal space does not exist: only the surfaces of self and object are experienced. Objects or events cannot be taken in or thought about since there is no inside: no mind capable of reverie in the object, nor a place in the self for phantasy, thought and memory. Objects are therefore like sheets of paper, with only a front and a back (Fano Cassese, 2018). Following Meltzer I would like to suggest that in the context of incest, two-dimensionality annihilates not only processes of internalization but also processes of projective identification. In addition to the fact that projective identification essentially demands three-dimensionality, in this process contents projected into the object are returned to the subject mixed with the object's containing qualities. But when the container itself is experienced as having malignant, contaminating qualities, as in the case of the incestuous object, the entire process of projective identification becomes an enactment of the primary incestuous scene and is unconsciously blocked.

Thus, the attack of the incestuous scene on thinking and language has a number of intertwined components: First, it creates a malignant ambiguity of concealing and revealing. This ambiguity constitutes an attack on the child's "function of translation", in Laplanche's terms, leading to an a priori refusal of any enigmatic quality. Second, it institutes a container/contained interaction in which thinking is experienced as enacting the primary threat, thus prompting in the child a rejection not just of certain specific thoughts, but of the very act of thinking. Third, the incestuous scene brings about an unconscious blockage of processes of projective identification: since the object is experienced as malignant, the contents that have been deposited in it cannot possibly be taken back as they have become contaminated with the object's malignant contents and qualities.

As a result of this multiple attack on thinking the infantile mind turns to two types of psychic organization characterized, as mentioned before, by their two-dimensionality. The first type attacks the container/contained interaction (both its intra- and interpersonal aspects) by means of a flattening of psychic life and a rejection of any sort of dream work or reverie; the second type attacks the container/contained interaction (both its intra- and interpersonal aspects) by adopting a pseudo-phallic position, allowing only one direction of psychic movement (from the inside outward), thus preventing any penetration. These two types of organization will now be illustrated by means of the two following clinical cases.

## The overall flattening of three-dimensionality

M., in her thirties and mother of one, applied to once-weekly psychotherapy about two and a half years ago because she wanted to "deepen her acquaintance with herself". As a child she suffered incest from her brother who was eight years older, a beloved brother who was a kind of father figure to her since her actual father was experienced as detached and absent. The incest, which went on approximately between ages 5 and 15, involved rubbing in the nude, anal penetration and coaxing her into joint masturbation. She doesn't talk much about her childhood, and when she does refer to events of that period it is mostly without words, using pantomime-like, silent gestures. Her world is divided into attackers and victims, including her own five years old son whom she sometimes experiences as a potential rapist. In the world she describes, things move mechanically from one extreme to another, never gaining volume or depth. Everything has the same horizontal pendulum-like quality: her partner may be the most caring and loving person on one occasion, while in our next session she may portray him as alienated and egotistical. She makes no effort to connect these different layers, and lacks any sense of how and why her experience of him shifts from one end to another. His various "characters" simply coexist in her mind separately, alongside each other, making no contact. A similar oscillation also marks her relations with her only son. In one session she may feel deeply attached to him, while in another she feels nothing but alienation and hostility.

This is far beyond an internalization of a perplexing "revolving" object (protecting her from harm at one moment while hurting her in the next): M. displays a chronic flattening associated with a resistance to and a dread of any kind of complexity. Whatever suggests layeredness or depth triggers huge anxiety in the face of which she simply disconnects or dissociates. Interpretations that are too nuanced have a way of passing her by, as though she doesn't hear them. She gets distracted, and while she blames her attention disorder, it is clear to me that what really prevents her from listening to these interpretations is that any nuanced, layered poetics immediately transforms into a poetics of suspicion, which puts an intolerable threat between us. Though she ostensibly wishes to gain more depth, her therapy (which she refuses to turn into analysis) remains stuck for the first two years in a concrete and superficial mode. She needs me (and is grateful when I oblige) to "get organized", "make order"—as she calls it, by which she means the moments in which we engage in the opposite of in-depth analytic work: this is when I help her turn chaos and complexity into something orderly, well-defined, which she can contain. At these moments I concretely assist her to recover the differences between right and wrong, logical and not logical, healthy and unhealthy. However, any interpretations that head in the opposite direction, i.e. invoke awareness of the layered texture of things—are rejected outright.

In the countertransference I feel extremely cautious. Since interpretation is bound to be experienced as an invasion or a trap, not only my words but the whole therapeutic setting is charged: whenever I let her stay a few more minutes, or positively respond to her request to change the time of the session, she reacts with anxiety. She says she feels guilty because she "squeezes" me for more time, but I sense that she is anxious because in her unconscious experience it is not clear enough whether the desire (for more time, for more closeness) is mine or hers. In that sense whenever I fulfill her wish, she may experience it as if she is the one who fulfilled mine. When I try to interpret in this direction she withdraws.

There is a constant movement between connection and alienation. This is enacted also in the body: when I say something that touches her she may respond: "I don't understand what you are saying but I am in tears, so it must be true". I feel in those moments that she is physically penetrated by my words, without allowing their meaning to enter her mind. I ask myself whether this can be understood as a kind of enactment of the primary incestuous scene, in which contents were ejaculated into her body in a manner that bypassed her mind.

One day she tells me that when her brother rubbed himself against her, mostly at night, she would often sing. When I ask what she sang, she repeats a song the same brother used to sing to her when she was afraid of the dark. Beyond the song's concrete function—which clearly helped to mobilize her brother as a warm and good object during these unbearable moments (even though the integration of his caring image and his abusive image was and remained for many years unattainable to her)—it also served as a barrier, enabling, to some extent, the same flattening she continues to use against any kind of complexity. She sang so that one voice would cover or drown out another; she sang so that the protective-paternal cadence would erase the sexual cadence from their interaction; she sang in order to re-install a split between good and evil and to protect her from their insufferable blending. As she tells me these things I realize that in her psychotherapy—which naturally causes contact with the "dark" elements of her mind—she uses the same method: she asks me to sing her the reassuring, comforting tune which restores order and calms her down, but rather than using it as a way in, she uses it as a way out, disconnecting through it from what she cannot face.

For years she would tell herself the narrative her brother taught her "without getting confused", because if she got confused (and put things the way she experienced them rather than the way he told them), things might appear—her brother warned her—"exactly the opposite of how they really were". In her brother's narrative, he touches her not to hurt her but to teach her how men act with little girls, so she will know how to defend herself when they try. It's his way of protecting her. It's only because he loves her so much that he wants her to experience it for the first time with him rather than with some stranger who just wants to use her. This way she'll learn about her body and know what she likes, and when she'll grow up and men will touch her, she won't make "beginners mistakes". Other girls, whose brothers don't teach them, are totally ignorant and then get hurt, but she will be the most clued up of all.

This twisted, perverse narrative fatally entangled M.'s ability to think what was going on. Presenting itself as a road map, this was a narrative that obliterated the roads and produced inversion, dissimulation and equivocation. The reason she kept quiet for years was because she knew that if she told, people might attack their hermetic dyad—a dyad which simultaneously and in a psychotic, ambiguous manner hurt her but also shielded her from feelings of guilt and shame.

This narrative chillingly illustrates the ambiguity of revealment and concealment which is the focus of this chapter. Pretending to produce meaning it actually upended what happened, removing one meaning in order to pour in another, all this by using a pseudo-logic which rendered the account hermetic, impenetrable to thinking. This is not merely a matter of the adult body forcing itself upon the child's body: what we witness here is an adult force of thinking imposing itself on the immature childish thinking in a way that attacks the most fundamental coordinates of that thinking. As a result of this violent use of pseudo-logic, contact with anything nuanced or layered reproduces and enacts, in M.'s unconscious experience, the threat of the ambiguous primal scene.

When, for instance, she tells me how she feared entering her empty home when returning from school as a child, and I suggest her fear may have been related not to the empty home but to what might be awaiting her there (her brother), she rejects that possibility and insists it was the builders at work nearby she feared. The possibility that she is splitting off a threat that is actually related to her brother—whom she experiences as protecting her from them—is at this point impossible for her to contemplate.

But what is striking in this situation, rather than the split-off contents or the partial object relations she entertains, is the way a flattening terror forces itself not only on her thinking but also on mine. Only with hindsight do I realize that what she has been telling me was not merely about her fear of entering the actual house where her brother might or might not be awaiting her but also about her dread of "entering her inner space", her inner world of phantasies and urges with which any contact was experienced as life threatening. It is the enigma whose messages she cannot "translate", the enigma whose translatability was attacked when invaded by an anti-metabolic element, in Lapanche's terms, that constitutes the threat due to which she always "stayed outside": outside the therapeutic process as well as outside herself. However, it wasn't only she who feared entering the empty house but me as well. My interpretations, too, have for a long time stuck close to the surface of her narrative, attempting the reconstruction of her conscious history while avoiding the possibility to set foot into the obscure territory of her unconscious historicity.

What was lacking in this therapeutic text was a type of volume related to the sediments of dream-work included in the layers of the waking texture. These exactly were the strata excluded from the en-counter with M. For a long time I felt as though I had internalized an incestuous object that put me under the same terror she lived with, and which made it wholly impossible to escape the surface of her narrative. As in the case with the narrative her brother had imposed on her, I, too, was concerned for a long time that what I said might be understood as "exactly the opposite of what it really was". I felt that my hands were tied, and that I didn't have the freedom which is the essence of psychoanalytic language and thinking.

Laplanche (1998) distinguishes two modalities of transference which he calls "filled-in" transference and "hollowed-out" transference: "The central place of transference results from the fact that the analyst adopts an attitude based on an ethics of refusal. By first denying himself knowledge, the analyst offers the patient a space, a "hollow" in which the latter may place either something "filled-in" or another "hollow" (Scarfone, 2013, p. 558). Filled-in transference consists in "the positive reproduction of forms of behavior, relationships and childhood im-agos" (Laplanche, 1989, p. 161 [1987, p. 157]); this is transference as it is commonly described, i.e., the repetition of archaic situations. In hollowed-out transference, however, "it is the childhood relationship that is repeated; it regains its enigmatic character" (ibid). Hollowed-out transference implies that "the enigmatic messages of childhood are reactivated, investigated and worked through thanks to the situation itself as it facilitates the return of the enigmatic and secondary revision" (ibid.). This situation thus confronts the patient with the enigma of the other, now embodied by the analyst: the patient, much like the infant, is confronted with the hollow, the open space where new translations of the enigma may issue, so that one is not doomed to sheer repetition of the same (Scarfone, 2013). In M.'s case the terror of incest was inflicted on both types of transference. Since both the archaic situations as well as the enigma of primary relations were traumatically contaminated, the transference relations remained locked in a narrow space delimited by two types of negation: the negation of reproducing the archaic situations and the negation of reviving the archaic enigma.

In contrast with these serious constraints on the actual transference and countertransference relationship, I found myself flooded—both during sessions and between them—by active reverie materials of a surprising intensity. In a sense, my own mind was stalling at the terror coming its way, forcing upon me an onslaught of unsolved enigmas, requests for translation, riddles to whose colorfulness and intensity no orderly logical sequence was adequate. M. appeared frequently in my dreams, at times as a child, then again as an adult woman, often located in a closed space and trying to forge a path to me or away from me. I did not understand how crucially important the intensity of these dreams or this dream-work was, until the day that M. herself brought her first dream. It was some time after the end of her second year of psychotherapy. In the dream she is locked into a narrow passage which has neither entrance nor exit. A kind of intestine, she says, whose two ends are tied. She has no associations concerning this image. The only thing she recalls is that they had something like that, a traditional Jewish dish, filled "kishke"—intestine—last Saturday.

Aware that the intestine resembles the male sexual organ, I didn't want to interpret the obvious, nor did I dare to cross the line of what she could bear. And so I asked about the feeling of no way out. M. said that it was similar, in a way, to that one time she tried to tell her mother something about what her brother was doing to her. She was not explicit, just cast about for words, stammering, to which her mother responded: "Oh, don't make a fuss, it's all natural". She remembers feeling suffocated in the small bathroom, and the impossibility of getting either out or in. As she says this, I recollect my dream of the night before. In that dream I am stuck in a narrow hallway leading to my own clinic, but the entrance to the clinic is blocked. Since there is no way out other than by entering the room, I understand that I will be unable to get out unless I manage somehow to get in. Then I wake up. At this point in the session I understand, with shocking intensity, that M. and I are locked in an intestine with both ends tied up.

The terror exercised by the past and the fear of reproducing it, made us withdraw from the possibility of anything new emerging between us. There is no way out of the therapeutic space, much like the intestine in her dream and the hallway in mine, simply because there is no way in. M. is imprisoned in a blocked intestine of thinking: she can neither digest nor expel, neither take in nor eject. Her thinking apparatus, and my analytic apparatus no less, "is tied at both ends".

Here a parasitic interaction occurs in which the contained crams the container with toxic material, while the container does not let the toxic material either be digested or evacuate (Ogden, 2003). Thinking, too, is an act of excretion. If M. expels the toxic material, the room will become smelly and dirty. If she doesn't, it may soil, perhaps destroy, her entire inner space. Finally I say: "The intestine is tied up at both ends. Opening one of them means to soil the outside. Not opening it means soiling the inside". To my surprise, M. replies: "Better to mess up the outside. Unless one of the ends gets untied—I will die". Then she starts crying. "I feel nauseous", she says, "just thinking of it. But also lighter". Even now I find it hard to describe the sense of relief that filled the room at that moment. As if something in the blocked intestine had opened up.

In a chapter dedicated to the trauma of incest, Bollas (1989) argues that when the father commits incest, development switches direction: instead of moving from the region of pure impulses to the territory of symbolization and sublimation, the girl is oriented away from symbolic domains to those of gratification of (and in) the concrete reality and the concrete body. This constitutes an attack not merely on the girl's body but also on her mind. When the father penetrates the domain of dreams and dreaming, he makes the dream an unsafe space, insufficiently protected from reality, i.e. insufficiently marked out as an internal space. This does not interfere just with the child's ability to fall asleep and dream, but also with her ability to evolve a separate mental life, and to experience processes of reverie (Bollas, 1989).

M.'s evolving ability to allow herself processes of reverie, dream work and dream life, expressed itself not only in the concrete dreams she began to bring in but also in her increased capacity to cope with vagueness, as well as with the enigmatic qualities of the therapeutic language. I understand, in retrospect, that the "storage" of the deeper layers of her thinking in the domain of my own reverie—eventually allowed for the intolerable materials to linger in thinking. As a result, it gradually became possible to trade the work of reconstructing a known past—against the capacity and freedom to dream the unknown.

## The pseudo-phallic position

Y., an opinionated young woman who experienced incestuous relations with her father in her early childhood, seeks analysis almost against her will, after repeatedly having been taken to task by her employer for her problematic attitude to her colleagues. Y. is not willing for anyone to interfere with anything she says or thinks. There's only one truth and she owns it. Others are "poor non-entities", "liars", "frauds", "cheats". Her discourse terrifies in its barren repetitiveness. Very rarely tears well up in her eyes, but she is quick to wipe them away and they are more like tears of rage than tears of pain. Rage, in contrast with pain, lacks a melancholy tone. It aims at the others, the violators, those who abandon, ignore, turn their backs, and it points at them like a weapon, never like a hand held out.

As a rule, she takes the depth out of all duality, complexity, or ambivalence. One can only enter one bond with her, and this bond has no room for an intersubjectivity in which one person can serve as a witness to the other. Instead she produces a horror show: facing her—well-organized, fluent, impeccable—one can only take the position of a silent spectator, passively taking in her statements. As far as she's concerned, others hate her because they fear the truth she exposes. That's why she's so alone. She may want to die—or to kill—but her own melancholy is inaccessible to her since it undergoes a sado-masochistic transformation into revenge. Instead of a work of mourning, she sets store by a fetishistic, vengeful ritual which leaves her not only isolated from others but also locked out of herself.

Y. is the only child of a literature professor who had incestuous relations with her throughout her early childhood. Among other things, he used to sit her on his lap, read her colorful stories, while rubbing against her, tickling her, tempting her to move and twist in a way that aroused him sexually. Her mother, who witnessed this usually from the kitchen, used to shout at him: "Leave her, she is your daughter, not your lover!" but did nothing to stop it.

She remembers how her father used to put her to bed, rubbing himself against her in a sexual manner while singing a German lullaby about an adult man who asks a little girl to "open her garden gate" and "do him a favor". The song revealed the truth but simultaneously served as a cover up: not just because pretending to sing a lullaby, the father was stimulating both himself and the child, but also because under the cover of truth (the lullaby's words) he actually erased the meaning of that truth: transforming it into something that was out there for all to hear, it became something that need not be revealed either to others or to herself.

Y., a gifted child who shared a poetic, sophisticated language with her father as a toddler, today, as a grown up, uses extremely rough speech. As far as she is concerned any metaphor is a lure. "People need to speak directly", she says, "without detours". And since psychoanalytic language is essentially metaphoric (using images and sometimes relating to abstract aspects of the mind as if they were bodily organs), Y. cannot stand most of the things I say. Whenever I dare to say something with a whiff of metaphor she feels betrayed and becomes violent. This has nothing to do with her capacity to understand what is said. It is the language itself that she cannot abide.

Her incapacity to bear complexity, neither as content nor as a form, is enacted in her attitude toward the setting, too: although I offered her four times a week analysis, to which she agreed—she refuses to lie on the couch. The couch for her is a symbol of complexity, of layeredness. It directs her inward, and this she cannot bear. Instead, she sits facing me, usually directing her gaze at my shoes. Only after more than a year is she occasionally able to look beyond me, through the window. I understand it as a gesture of faith, a sign she trusts that I won't take advantage of her "turning inward" in order to use her for my satisfaction.

The analytic challenge with Y. was to restore even the most primitive processes of projective identification: to enable her to "take back" contents that she deposited in me without feeling invaded and contaminated by them, without experiencing them as violent "gang members" out to conquer her inner space.

Y. offers a striking example of the defensive pseudo-phallic position: the tactic is one of continuous ejection by way of a defense against any possibility of penetration or internalization. Bollas (1989) suggested that in the case of incestuous relations between father and daughter the girl sometimes creates a kind of phallic prosthesis, an artificial limb that replaces symbolic thinking with an artificial mold that forecloses all sorts of vital containment. Y. refuses to form any sort of mental container which can be invaded. Hence she holds on to the surface of thinking in a grandiose way, avoiding any dialogue which would essentially give access to otherness. Since every penetration contaminates—all types of penetration meet with refusal.

After almost a year of analysis, Y. came to a session wearing a raincoat zipped all the way up to her chin. She sat down in the chair facing me, dripping wet, and started, as usual, to fire furious sentences. She was furious about the rain, she was furious about the weather forecast which predicted a nice spring day, she was furious with the bus driver who, driving right through a puddle, sprayed her with water and mud, and she was furious with me: because I run a clinic near a very busy street, she is forced, on her way to me, to brush against all kinds of violent characters, "...who make me lose any wish to talk about myself, because it is them who actually need analysis, not me".

Whatever I said infuriated her, and any interpretation bounced—as happened very often in our sessions—against her comment that I obviously didn't understand her, never had and never would. At some point during this attack I found myself thinking of a jazz performance I attended some years back, when the pianist improvised on the rhythm of a speaking human voice. Maybe it was my frustration and despair, but suddenly, inspired by this recollection, I stopped listening to what Y. was saying and took in the music of her voice alone. To my surprise, and unlike the repetitive subject matter, her voice was colorful. At times it blasted, but there were also moments when a melancholic quality slipped in, almost introverted, and in those moments it wasn't really clear who she was firing at: me or herself.

"Y.", I said, "you're shooting every which way, but when I stop worrying about your rage, what I hear is that you're stuck in your fury like in a cage: you have no idea how to hold out a hand, and you don't believe there's any hand out there that might take yours. You ignore my words the same way you cold-shoulder those pushy types outside, they scare you, my words, as if they were traps put in your way to weaken you. But then you are left without them and without me, and that loneliness only worsens the anger and the frustration, as well as the urge to destroy everything, including both of us".

She looked me in the eye, softly, for the first time in months: "So what are you saying?" she asked quietly. "I am saying that I know you're scared to death about letting me in. I know you don't believe that I will not use any opening you make for me in order to hurt you. But I also know that when you dismiss me, you turn away not just from me but also from a part of yourself. And perhaps what you need is for me not to let you continue turning away from it".

This was a first step toward a change that took months to unfold. It wasn't a linear process. Changes in a traumatic fabric cannot be linear since they carry the fragmentary qualities of the fabric itself. What I understand now is that the musical recollection here—like the recollected dream in the previous clinical illustration—served to unconsciously restore polyphony to the two-dimensional texture of the analytic relationship. It was my way of unconsciously reclaiming the freedom to shift between different vocal layers and depths, rather than being frozen into a position of "passive absorption". It was also my way of inviting her to replace what seemed to be a blind evacuation of any contact with her interior—with an access to her own lost polyphony of voice and language.

## From ambiguity to ambivalence

Bleger (1973) postulates that ambiguity is characteristic of the most primitive organization of the personality. To situate the concept of ambiguity, he writes, we need to refer to two other concepts. One is ambivalence, which classically denotes the possibility of love and hate for the same object at the same time. The other is the mechanism of "divalence" which, through splitting, brings it about that one separately loves and hates two different objects (Bleger, 2017). This enables one to avoid the conflict of ambivalence, and experience each feeling with a different object as if there were no connection between these feelings or between these objects. To these two concepts, Bleger adds ambiguity. In its classic definition, ambiguity is "what may be understood in different ways or what is imprecise or indefinite":

> We say someone is ambiguous when he is "variable, irresolute, changeable"; when he alternately shows varying trends, affects, attitudes or behavior, which, though contradictory or mutually exclusive to the observer, are not to him who persists in an indefinite or undetermined state. (1973a, p. 455)

While divalence is characteristic of the paranoid-schizoid position, and ambivalence marks the depressive position, ambiguity is typical of the most primitive mode of mental functioning, prior to the paranoid-schizoid position. Bleger suggests that while in the states of ambivalence and of divalence the subject experiences the contradictions between good and bad (as different qualities of the same object in ambivalence, or as different qualities of different objects in divalence), in the state of ambiguity there is no experience of contradiction, since the qualities are not experienced as sufficiently distinct to afford such a sense.

One may think of the confusion the language of incest creates as turning what should have been a healthy ambivalence into a malignant ambiguity. As a result of the ambiguity of the incestuous scene—In which the differentiation between good and bad, pain and pleasure, fantasy and reality and child and adult is so blurred—both thinking and language turn into a territory of pseudo-logic in which contradictory narratives can coexist freely and uninterruptedly.

In M.s' case, this pseudo-logic was reflected in the narrative her brother "planted" in her. This narrative transformed a story of abuse into a story of rescue as it demolished any coordinate for thinking it differently. In Y.'s case, as borne out by the lullaby her father used to sing to her, the story simultaneously exposed and hid what was inflicted on her, and thereby made any possibility of her discovering what had occurred—redundant. Ambiguous language did not merely make it impossible for these two girls to think about specific contents. It was generalized in them to a comprehensive attack on any kind of container/contained interaction, and therefore on both thinking and dreaming. The terror the ambiguous language inflicted on their thinking triggered a "counter-terror". This terror, in order to avoid both contamination and penetration, imposed a two-dimensional agenda on all regions of thought.

We can think of the psychoanalytic process as pursuing the chance to create a shift from the ambiguous territory of (non)thinking in which contradicting narratives coexist—to the territory of ambivalence, where different aspects of the same narrative are contained in the narrating voice. But the road leading there is extremely complex. This complexity is related to the fact that the psychoanalytic scene itself can be experienced as ambiguous due to the structural contamination it elicits between past and present, inside and outside, transference relations and concrete relations. Where the initial language carries a malignant ambiguity, and eliminates the possibility of translation rather than stimulating translation, the whole analytic scene may transform, in the patient's experience, into a scene of violent penetration of the analyst's desire into the patient's mental space. In this scene, the analyst's enigma, rather than activating creativity and curiosity, poses a threat, and the question "What does the analyst want from me?" becomes a riddle with only one answer: the analyst's desire which the patient must satisfy. In other words, the inherent enigma of the analytic relationship, the "ethical seduction" (Shetrit-Vatine, 2018), becomes a barrier which rather than activating processes of thinking violently blocks them.

The psychoanalytic scene poses a primary demand to the patient to "open up" (to associations, to fantasies, to transference relations and repetitions). But where in a patient's unconscious phantasy every such opening is bound to be violently penetrated by the other's thoughts and interpretations, psychoanalytic work is experienced as severely precarious. This is where the preliminary work on the preconditions for analytic dialogue, much before beginning the analytic work with the actual contents, is so indispensable. This requires recognition of the unique meaning the essential psychoanalytic factors have for patients who are incest victims: recognition of their experience that every interpretation is an invasion via the openings of thought; recognition that the psychoanalytic environment itself is opaque and ambiguous; recognition of the experience that any new content threatens irreversible contamination and expropriation.

At stake is the restoration of the patient's function of translation. The interpretation of the essential factors of analysis aims precisely at this function. Rather than dealing with content, they deal with the unconscious implications of the analytic language and the analytic scene regarding the patient's ability to translate, illuminating their unconscious charging. The purpose of such interpretations is to reactivate the translation process that will constitute in its turn a platform for the analytic scene to emerge.

But these formal interpretations are not enough in order for deep analytic work to occur. In addition to the necessary platform they provide, the analyst, through his or her reverie work, needs to offer what interpretations cannot reach, namely to preserve a polyphonic internal space whose layers dilute the flattening mechanisms, and which holds onto what the elimination mechanisms have cast out. Whether in sleep or awake, the analyst's dream-work serves as a thinking enclave which hosts what has been banished from the patient's thinking as well as from the analytic discourse.

Only once polyphony is brought back into the here and now of the transference and countertransference, will analysis be able to shift from the compulsive repetition of "the death of language" (Lazar, 2017) to a mode of witnessing (Amir, 2016) which marks language as both a way out and a way in.

## References

Amir, D. (2016). When Language Meets the Traumatic Lacuna: The Metaphoric, the Metonymic and the Psychotic modes of testimony. *Psychoanalytic Inquiry, 36*(8), 620–632.

Amir, D. (2017). Screen Confessions: A Current Analysis of Nazi Perpetrators' 'Newspeak'. *Psychoanalysis, Culture & Society, 23*(1), 97–114.

Bion, W. (1959). Attacks on Linking. *International Journal of Psycho-Analysis, 40*, 308–315.

Bion, W. (1962a). *Learning from Experience*. New York, NY: Basic Books.

Bion, W. (1962b). The Psycho-Analytic Study of Thinking. *International Journal of Psycho-Analysis, 43*, 306–310.

Bion, W. (1970). *Attention and Interpretation*. London: Tavistock.

Bleger, J. (1973). Ambiguity: A Concept of Psychology and Psychopathology. In S. Arieti (Ed.). *The World Biennial of Psychiatry and Psychotherapy*. New York, NY: Basic Books, Vol. 2, pp. 453–470.

Bleger, J. (2013 [1967]). *Symbiosis and Ambiguity: A Psychoanalytic Study* (New Library of Psychoanalysis, trans., Rogers S., Bleger L., Churcher J.). In Churcher J. & Bleger L. (Eds.) . London: Routledge.

Bleger, L. (2017). José Bleger's Thinking about Psychoanalysis. *The International Journal of Psychoanalysis*, *98*(1), 145–169.

Bollas, C. (1989). *Forces of Destiny: Psychoanalysis and Human Idiom*. London: Free Association Books.

Fano Cassese, S. (2018). *Introduction to the Work of Donald Meltzer*. London and New York: Routledge.

Ferenczi, S. (1949). Confusion of the Tongues Between the Adults and the Child—(The Language of Tenderness and of Passion)1. *International Journal of Psycho-Analysis*, *30*, 225–230.

Laplanche, J. (1989[1987]). *New Foundations for Psychoanalysis* (trans. D. Macey). Oxford: Blackwell.

Laplanche, J. (1998). Transference: Its Provocation by the Analyst. In J. Fletcher (Ed.). *Essays on Otherness*. London: Routledge.

Lazar, R. (2017). Trying to Conceive the Inconceivable. In R. Lazar (Ed.). *Talking about Evil*. London: Routledge, pp. 200–217.

Lyotard, J.-F. (1989). *The Differend: Phrases in Dispute*. (Theory and History of Literature, Vol. 46), (Trans. G. Van Den Abbeele). Minneapolis: University of Minnesota Press.

Meltzer, D. (1975). Dimensionality as a parameter of mental functioning: its relation to narcissistic organization. In D. Meltzer, J. Bremner, S. Hoxter, D. Weddell, & I. Wittenberg (Eds.). *Explorations in Autism*. Strath Tay: Clunie Press, pp. 223–238.

Ogden, T. H. (2003). On Not Being Able to Dream. *International Journal of Psychoanalysis*, *84*(2003), 17–30.

Scarfone, D. (2013). A Brief Introduction to the Work of Jean Laplanche. *International Journal of Psycho-Analysis*, *94*(3), 545–566.

Shetrit-Vatine, V. (2018). *The Ethical Seduction of the Analytic Situation: The Feminine-Maternal Origins of Responsibility for the Other*. London & New York: Routledge.

# Chapter 3

# The two sleeps of Orlando: gender transition as caesura or cut

Gender dichotomy may well be the most primary dichotomy internalized in human thinking. It acts as a prototype for all the later dichotomies, inaugurating, one might say, dichotomous thinking in general—first within the imaginary of the parent who holds the soon to be born infant in his or her mind, and later within the mind of the infant itself. This chapter focuses on the conditions which enable the establishment of a dialectic and unsaturated gender space—one that allows both a concrete and a fantasized creative mobility between the two gender poles—versus the conditions which generate a polar, saturated, gender dichotomous stagnation and stasis.

One of the most famous literary expressions of the idea of an unsaturated gender space is Virginia Woolf's *Orlando* ([1928] 1949). This is perhaps her most eccentric book: a clever and ironic "wink", as Haim Pesach (2007) writes in the introduction to the Hebrew translation, a moment of mischief in this brilliant and tragic author's oeuvre. The novel deals with the relationships between men and women and gender identity through the story of a young man who, after a long deep sleep, turns into a woman and continues to lead a life of romance and love for over 300 years.

Twice in the course of the book, Orlando falls into what may be a sleep or a mysterious coma. The first episode occurs when he is abandoned by his girlfriend and falls into a deep dissociative sleep to overcome his heartbreak. In the second sleep, somewhat reminiscent of Genesis' scene of God's creation of Eve from Adam's body ("And the LORD God caused a deep sleep to fall upon Adam, and he slept: and he took one of his ribs, and closed up the flesh instead thereof";

DOI: 10.4324/9781003194071-3

Genesis, 2:21), Orlando transforms from a man into a woman. I would like to begin by identifying the different characteristics of these two sleeps of Orlando, and subsequently connect them to two types of gender crossing: gender crossing (or gender mobility) which enables the transformation of "gender excess", as opposed to gender crossing that is in itself an acting-out of this excess rather than an act of transformation.

Orlando's first sleep is described as follows:

> One June morning—it was Saturday the 18th—he failed to rise at his usual hour, and when his groom went to call him he was found fast asleep. Nor could he be awakened. He lay as if in a trance, without perceptible breathing; and though dogs were set to bark under his window; cymbals, drums, bones beaten perpetually in his room; a gorse bush put under his pillow; and mustard plasters applied to his feet, still he did not wake, take food, or show any sign of life for seven whole days. On the seventh day he woke at his usual time (a quarter before eight, precisely) and turned the whole posse of caterwauling wives and village soothsayers out of his room, which was natural enough; but what was strange was that he showed no consciousness of any such trance, but dressed himself and sent for his horse as if he had woken from a single night's slumber. Yet some change, it was suspected, must have taken place in the chambers of his brain, for though he was perfectly rational and seemed graver and more sedate in his ways than before, he appeared to have an imperfect recollection of his past life. He would listen when people spoke of the great frost or the skating or the carnival, but he never gave any sign, except by passing his hand across his brow as if to wipe away some cloud, of having witnessed them himself. When the events of the past six months were discussed, he seemed not so much distressed as puzzled, as if he were troubled by confused memories of some time long gone or were trying to recall stories told him by another. [...] But if sleep it was, of what nature, we can scarcely refrain from asking, are such sleeps as these? Are they remedial measures—trances in which the most galling memories, events that seem likely to cripple life for ever, are brushed with a dark wing which rubs their harshness

off and gilds them, even the ugliest and basest, with a lustre, an incandescence? Had Orlando, worn out by the extremity of his suffering, died for a week, and then come to life again? (pp. 63–64)

This allegorical, partly ironic description, is in fact one of dissociative detachment. During his seven-day sleep, Orlando sheds his painful memories, and when he wakes up he can resume his life supposedly from the point where it was interrupted. Yet this is a mechanical, somewhat hollow continuity which does not enable him to maintain a vivid continuity regarding himself or his life. In effect he loses the "function of the inner witness" (Amir, 2012), or the function of the "biographer" as Woolf calls it throughout the book: the inner function that enables a person to be in touch with experience and at the same time deviate from it and reflect on it. Orlando, who, from the moment he wakes up, lacks the ability to bear witness to the story of his life as his own story, can only take one of two positions: he may allow himself to experience the unbearable but at the risk of suffering another collapse. Alternatively, he may bear witness to his story as if it were not his, by holding on to the facts without an emotional connection to the experience, and thus stay alive at the cost of losing his liveliness. Either way his mental existence remains incomplete, and this is his condition until he undergoes the second transformation that allows him renewed access to the memories lost during the first sleep.

Orlando's second sleep is described in the following words:

Next morning, the Duke, as we must now call him, was found by his secretaries sunk in profound slumber amid bed clothes that were much tumbled. [...] No suspicion was felt at first, as the fatigues of the night had been great. But when afternoon came and he still slept, a doctor was summoned. He applied remedies which had been used on the previous occasion, plasters, nettles, emetics, etc., but without success. [...] Morning and evening they watched him, but, save that his breathing was regular and his cheeks still flushed their habitual deep rose, he gave no sign of life. Whatever science or ingenuity could do to waken him they did. But still he slept. (pp. 121–122)

As in the previous sleep, Orlando wakes up after seven days:

> He stretched himself. He rose. He stood upright in complete
> nakedness before us, and while the trumpets pealed Truth! Truth!
> Truth! we have no choice left but confess—he was a woman. [...]
> Orlando had become a woman—there is no denying it. But in
> every other respect, Orlando remained precisely as he had been.
> The change of sex, though it altered their future, did nothing
> whatever to alter their identity. Their faces remained, as their
> portraits prove, practically the same. His memory—but in future
> we must, for convention's sake, say "her" for "his", and "she" for
> "he"—her memory then, went back through all the events of her
> past life without encountering any obstacle. Some slight haziness
> there may have been, as if a few dark drops had fallen into the
> clear pool of memory; certain things had become a little dimmed;
> but that was all. [...] Many people, taking this into account, and
> holding that such a change of sex is against nature, have been at
> great pains to prove (1) that Orlando had always been a woman,
> (2) that Orlando is at this moment a man. Let biologists and
> psychologists determine. It is enough for us to state the simple
> fact; Orlando was a man till the age of thirty, when he became a
> woman and has remained so ever since. (pp. 126–128)

Orlando's second sleep, unlike the preceding one, culminates in a real
transformation. But this transformation from man to woman does not
come at the cost of dissociation. Not only doesn't it block access to
memories, it paves a way to the memories blocked by the first sleep's
dissociation. The difference between Orlando's first and second sleep is
that while the former erected a barrier between him and his previous life,
the latter enables him to maintain who he was together with who she is,
that is, to integrate the man and the woman within one speaking person:
"The change of sex, though it altered their future, did nothing whatever
to alter their identity" (ibid, p. 127). Thus, he becomes not only "she" but
also "they"—that is, the third person plural, which includes both man
and woman, past and present, interior and exterior in a consecutive and
continuous manner. In this context, the allusion to Genesis' creation of
Eve out of Adam's body is interesting. In the biblical episode two separate entities are created whose dichotomous nature, once constituted,

allows no going back. Virginia Woof, by contrast, reverts the dichotomous scene to its pre-dichotomous state by hinting that since the two identities originated from one body, they will always contain each other somehow, with varying degrees of balance. Both of Orlando's sleeps occur as a reaction to his encounter with excess. In the case of the first sleep, this is an excess of pain related to his beloved's abandonment. In the case of the second sleep, an excess of admiration is showered upon him which reaches its hysteric peak on the evening prior to his falling asleep: "Women shrieked. A certain lady, who was said to be dying for love of Orlando, seized a candelabra and dashed it to the ground" (ibid, p. 120). However, while the first sleep was a way to create dissociation of excess—the role of the second sleep is to transform it.

### Bion 1977

Bion's notion of the "caesura" (1989) contains both a break and continuity at the same time. A break beyond which there is no continuity is a cut rather than a caesura. Bion situates the caesura between the pre-catastrophic state and the post-catastrophic state of change, treating it not as a static point in space or time but rather as a richly dynamic space itself: "It is in course of transit, in the course of changing from one position to another that these people seem to be most vulnerable—as, for example, during adolescence or latency" (Bion, [1977] 1989, p. 53). p. 53). However, this vulnerability is precisely why the state of caesura has the richest potential for change. Bion contrasts the dividing of the world into mutually exclusive polar states—with the state in which two different views or perspectives function together in a productive dialectical, caesura-like manner (Aharoni and Bergstein, note 48 in the annotated translation to Hebrew). Development always relies on keeping different views in a non-saturated state, thus avoiding the fixation of the components of consciousness in a stasis which does not allow them to absorb new meanings. In this context, an important question is whether we formulate gender crossing in terms of caesura or in terms of a cut, or even more precisely: under which conditions should gender crossing be formulated in terms of caesura, and under which in terms of a cut?

As said, gender dichotomy is probably the most primary dichotomy internalized in human thinking. As with any dichotomy, it may collapse into a state of saturation, becoming fixated and allowing for only a miniscule degree, if any, of transformability; alternatively, it may remain unsaturated and in this sense contain movement, richness and layered meanings. When does gender dichotomy become a rich dialectic, as opposed to being constituted as a saturated excess, that is, as a dichotomy whose poles are not only distinct but also mutually exclusive?

An excess of saturated gender dichotomy forms under conditions that encourage saturated divisions. The propensity for saturated divisions may be innate or acquired, and is always related to an anxiety of ambiguity and the need to defend oneself through rigid thinking against the unexpected and the impermanent. In most cases, this propensity for saturated divisions is a general inclination of thinking which is not solely related to gender dichotomy, but it becomes especially charged in children who do not find themselves at the socially "expected" end of the gender dichotomy. In such cases, the tension between primary gender ambiguity and the social pressure for saturated dichotomy might evolve into a forced need to situate oneself on one gender pole, losing the freedom to experience (even in fantasy) movement between both poles. Where gender categories do not serve thinking but rather block it, children whose primary gender experience is ambiguous might feel trapped in a saturated dichotomy in which they cannot find their place.

In his article "The Other Room and Poetic Space" (1998), Ronald Britton develops the notion of the "other room" as the space of imagination and fiction. He suggests that the other room emerges as the subject imagines the parents' intercourse rather than observes their actual sexual relations. It concerns the unwitnessed primal scene rather than the actual one: the one we have imagined as happening in our absence and which exists only in our imagination, thereby becoming a space for fiction. Unlike Winnicott, who defined the transitional phenomenon as the psychological space arising from the relations between infant and mother, and hence situated between "me" and "not me", Britton argues that the creative space emanates from the internal triangular dynamic. Similar to Melanie Klein (1924) and Otto Rank (1915) who argued that the origins of the theatrical stage are in the imaginary location of the parental sexual act, Britton claims that there is a "primal romantic couple", a "phantasised ideal, super-sexual parental couple", consisting of mythical figures, a kind of primal Adam and Eve, who are "the stars of the screen and the objects of endless media voyeurism". Expelled from Heaven, we are compelled, as non-participating observers, to imagine *their* Paradise. That Paradise becomes our other room, forever unfulfilled, accompanied with the pain of longing (Britton, 1998, pp. 122–123).

Borrowing the terms "this room" and "the other room" from the field of poetic creativity to apply them to the field of gender, I would like to suggest that when gender becomes a saturated object it is exactly this ability to create movement between "this room" of actual gender, and "the other room" of the phantasmatic gender, that sustains damage. The possibility of establishing a rich and layered gender space crucially depends on the creative movement between this room and the other room, without each negating the other. When this is possible, even a child whose initial gender experience is ambiguous and layered will feel that s/he can creatively move between the gender poles without this mobility (in both its concrete and non-concrete aspects) posing a threat. Such movement between the different gendered spaces is, one may say, an integrated movement including all rooms, as well as the areas of overlap and interface between them, within one house, that is, within one self.

In my book *On the Lyricism of the Mind* (Routledge, 2016) I suggested a "lyrical dimension" of mental space, which is in charge of the integration of two experiential/perceptual modes: the continuous mode, which perceives the world as predictable, intelligible and logical—and the emergent mode which perceives the world as unpredictable, inexplicable and constantly changing. The integration of these two modes of experience, which Bion (1970) originally identified as constituting the container/contained interaction, yields the mind's capacity to presuppose constancy and continuity on the one hand, and to tolerate considerable deviations from them without losing one's sense of identity and biography, on the other hand. If we formulate the interaction between the emergent and the continuous principles of the self in Bion's (1970) terms we may suppose that wherever the interaction between the emergent and the continuous is parasitic in nature or takes the form of a "malignant containment" (Britton, 1998, p. 28), one of two things might happen: the continuous self may smother the emergent self, leaving the latter no space for movement or development, or alternatively, the emergent self might stretch the continuous self beyond its breaking point, crashing through its boundaries. Bion (1970) argued that the sense of catastrophe that attends such an interaction between the emergent and the continuous is related to the fact that the psychic space is unable to supply an experience of constancy beyond change, a constancy which is the primary condition for change. When the continuous principle prevails, the psychic space becomes lacking in depth and resonance, while when the emergent principle takes over, the psychic space turns into a terrifying nightmare. If, by contrast, the interaction is compatible, integration may occur, inaugurating what I call the lyrical dimension of the psychic space. The emergent is the force that preserves things in their unsaturated condition, whereas the continuous is the saturated state. The more fertile the interaction between the two, the more likely one is to experience oneself as owning a historical and biographical continuum on the one hand, and as being a singular individual whose creativity is allowed to interrupt this continuum, on the other.

"Gender excess" can also be formulated in terms of the relationship between the continuous and the emergent: for example, an excess of a "continuous gender experience" as opposed to an "emergent gender experience" could damage the possibility of establishing a "gender space" in which the continuous and the emergent entertain fertile dialectic relations. On the other hand, an excess of emergent gender experience, in which every shift threatens to change the deep nucleus of identity, may undermine the possibility of a congruent relationship between the two poles of gender dialectic (the actual and the phantasmatic). Gender is always in the process of emerging. Yet every emergence needs a continuous container for its forcefulness and volatility. When there is a "continuous" gender that can contain the various gender emergences in a way that doesn't force the self to undergo a catastrophic identity change—"a gender space" is created. However, where the continuous (which manifests itself, for example, in the a-priori propensity toward saturated dichotomies) is too fragile and rigid, and its encounter with the volatile and powerful emergent threatens breakdown, parasitical relations may form between the actual and the phantasmatic gender, resulting in anxiety which further builds up fragility and rigidness. Whether these parasitical relations end in confinement within the original gender or lead to a concrete sex change procedure, they share the same parasitic quality that resists transformation. In this sense, even if they lead to gender crossing, it is a "saturated crossing", one with the characteristics of a cut rather than a caesura; one in which the new gender demands ongoing maintenance on account of other areas of experience and thought, and, above all, one that enables no free mobility to the "other (previous) gender", which has now, in retrospect, become an ostracized and forbidden territory. Since saturated objects are characterized not only by rigidness and lack of transformability but also by fragility, the more saturated the object, the more it is at risk regarding any movement or change. In gender crossing, this fragility is at times manifested in the extreme subjugation to the new gender's stereotypical characteristics, representing a different version of the same saturated gender dichotomy which was the source of the suffering in the first place. One form this kind of saturated crossing may take is the refusal to look back at one's childhood photo albums, much like the refusal to mention one's previous name or to somehow otherwise contain one's previous identity in the new one. This refusal creates a defensive split between the different parts of one's life as well as the life of those surrounding them, parts whose inclusion in the continuous sequence of life and identity is of paramount importance.

Quinodoz (1998), who describes the analysis of Simone, a trans woman, writes in this context: "Simone complained of having "forgotten" her pre-surgery past and, in particular, the feelings that belonged to that period of her life" (ibid, p. 95). Further on she writes:

> What she was in fact doing was unconsciously rejecting her past—and it seemed to me that this aspect [...] did indeed fall within the purview of analysis. Without analysis, I could not see how Simone could ever become reconciled with a part of herself she thought she hated. In my view, she could not readily achieve a sense of inner cohesion and personal unity without coming to terms with the first half of her life. (Ibid, p. 99)

In such cases, it is important to think of psychotherapy or psychoanalysis as a process that encourages the possibility to contain the myriad shades of gender in the new gender rather than forego them. The distinction between pathology and growth in relation to gender crossing has to do with the question whether it is an act that undermines the saturated areas of thinking and experience, or is itself an enactment of this saturation. When gender (old or new) becomes an addictive subjugating object in itself, crossing becomes a saturated state that obstructs development rather than enabling it. This could of course be a temporary state, a natural result of anxiety, expressing the obsessive hold of what is still experienced as transient, threatened and unattainable, but it is important to expect that with time a person will be able to relate to the new gender with the same degree of flexibility and freedom that we would expect of him or her when relating, in an intact situation of a priori congruence, to their original gender. Treatment, in the case of gender crossing, must therefore focus on establishing a continuum between the identities and an integration between the different states of psyche and soma, rather than maintaining a split between them. To return to Orlando, one can think of analytic work with gender-crossing in terms of the second transformative sleep, which enabled integration, while being careful not to encourage forms of cut as manifested in the first sleep's dissociative rift.

Quinodoz (1998, p. 99) distinguishes between gender crossing deriving from a very early experience of being "imprisoned" within the wrong actual gender, as opposed to gender crossing deriving from unprocessed hatred toward the actual gender, not because it contradicts the subject's experience but because it arouses psychotic anxieties. Perhaps the distinction should not refer to the conscious and unconscious reasons for gender crossing but rather to the level of their symbolization. Certain instances of crossing are indeed related, as the case below bears out, to a concrete or imagined significant object that becomes a saturated object, and the identification with which becomes malignant. When this occurs, gender crossing might be a psychotic–fetishistic expression of the wish to become that very other, a wish that dangerously and deceptively hides, through a possible physical transformation, a psychic transformation that failed to take place.

## From cleft lip to cleft tongue

Dan, 29 years old, seeks psychotherapy in the midst of a sex change procedure. After approximately two years of hormonal treatment, he turns to me for consultation since he feels that the psychiatrist who has been treating him is "pushing" him to complete the transition, whereas Dan does not feel ready for it. He is terribly anxious and cannot explain why now, of all times, a moment before his planned surgery, he suddenly hesitates. Dan is a twin brother to Anne. The twins were born to relatively old parents (both in their forties) after years of fertility treatments and painful miscarriages. From the moment they were born, Dan recounts, there was a division of roles between them. Anne was a beautiful, fragile and sickly girl who attracted a lot of attention and evoked great concern. Dan, on the other hand, was a chubby and robust baby, healthy and lively, but since he was born with a cleft lip his face was, at least in his own opinion, "damaged" compared to Anne's face. He remembers how for years—even after the aesthetic defect was surgically corrected by two successive plastic operations—people would avert their eyes, "as if searching for a more comfortable place to rest them on". That more comfortable place was Anne's pretty face. Although Dan was in every way a clever and talented boy, he felt that he was living in her shadow, or more accurately, in her light. He always felt that he must protect her, yet he remembers feeling painfully exposed when he was not by her side. He describes people's gazes accosting him whenever Anne was not with him, and her face could not serve as his refuge, as intolerable and persecutory.

The relations between brother and sister were symbiotic in many ways, including early experiences of joint masturbation and sharing everything they owned: toys, clothes, food. When Anne was diagnosed with celiac disease, Dan too stopped eating the foods she was forbidden to eat. When Dan suffered insults from fellow players in his football team Anne ripped pictures of herself in the team uniform from the walls of her room. This symbiosis was not without a price. They had very few friends who were not shared; their attachment to one another limited their areas of interest; and above all, Dan recounts, their closeness left out their parents. They felt that all they needed was each other. Except for their physical care neither of them remembers their parents having a significant role in their concrete or emotional lives. It seems as if, very early on, the parents gave up on any attempt to penetrate their children's symbiotic dyad.

Dan remembers himself, already at an early age, jealous of Anne's beauty and wanting to be like her. Most of all, he envied her face.

While he experienced his own face as mutilated, hers was the ideal face that he could or should have had. He remembers standing next to her by the mirror, looking at her reflection instead of at his own. He also remembers a fantasy about his face having been mutilated during their birth (and not prior to it, as it actually was) and believing his cleft upper lip to be the result of his having sacrificed his face in order to let Anne be born whole and unharmed.

Dan recalls experiencing the words he was trying to utter as "spilling out of his mouth": "every word was accompanied by spitting, I couldn't articulate a single word without it coming with something physical in the form of spit, or if I had been eating—chewed food that would spill out along with the words". He remembers many social occasions on which he would let Anne complete his sentences since it was more convenient for him "not to use his mouth", and since "she always knew what [he] intended to say anyway". Thus, words constituted somatic objects rather than symbolic ones. This bears a huge significance, as I will discuss later, when it comes to Dan's decision to undergo the physical transformation which in many ways substituted for his incapacity to symbolize.

Anne seemed to have served as Dan's perfect imaginary image. He remembers feeling at a very early age that since Anne was born a girl she had somehow appropriated what should have been his: the beauty, the delicateness, the caring she received—all these were attributed to her being a girl rather than to her being who she was. Dan recalls his envious passion for everything she had: her clothes, her makeup accessories. In her wardrobe closet there were several dresses and shirts she bought and kept especially for him, pretending they were hers. He detested his body, which he experienced as cumbersome and damaged, and the early signs of puberty only added to his abhorrence. He fell in love with girls, but felt that he loved them as a girl and not as a boy. He wanted them to caress his hair, to touch his breasts. His sexual fantasies were never related to penetration but rather to friction, and in masturbation he always visualized his genital as a female genital rubbing against another female genital. The few sexual experiences he had were experiences in which he masturbated against a woman's body without penetrating her. His sexual wish was to "come on her" and not to "come inside her", he repeatedly mentioned. This phrasing might hint at the aggression, envy and hatred toward women (who for him were all extensions of Anne) concealed behind his desire to become a woman. This hatred may also explain the anxiety that arose during the process of preparing for sex-change surgery, which I describe further on.

The symbiotic twinship with Anne along with the critical physical difference between them created an inner environment of splitting: her perfect face as opposed to his damaged face, the love that she aroused as opposed to the aversion and embarrassment he aroused, at least in his own experience—all these were attributed to the gender dichotomy, turning it into a simultaneously rigid and extremely fragile one. When he reached the age of 18 he began to speak openly about his wish to undergo sex change. His parents reacted with "shocked alienation or alienated shock", as he put it, but nevertheless supported the process. In the course of it, however, misgivings began to emerge. Dan felt he could not find himself in his new body (which due to the hormone treatment was beginning to show feminine characteristics). He did not want to return to his old body, which he detested, but did not feel "at home" either in the new body he was developing. Even as a woman he still felt awkward and damaged compared to Anne; he wanted to be as pretty as she, but discovered that in actuality he was not going to become a prettier woman than the man he had previously been. Gradually the therapy sessions revealed that his unconscious phantasy was not to be a woman, but to be Anne herself. She was the object of his admiration and passion, and the process he had begun was a process whose purpose was not to join her but to be her, perhaps even to replace her.

Another aspect, emerging from Dan's dreams, was related to mutilation. As I previously mentioned, Dan's fantasy was that his face had been mutilated in order to allow Anne to be born flawlessly. Now, instead of experiencing the gender change procedures as remedial, he felt them as "adding mutilation to mutilation". In one of his dreams he is lying on the operating table. One of his legs is apparently longer than the other, and the purpose of the operation, so he is told by the doctors, is to shorten the longer leg which will enable him to walk without limping. During the operation, however, it is his short leg that is mistakenly shortened, and he completely loses his ability to walk. I understand this dream as touching upon Dan's immense anxiety around the changes in his body: the surgery, meant to fix what he had experienced as an a priori failure, was revealed in the dream as likely to bring about an even bigger and more irrevocable failure. The longed for surgery reflecting his wish to undo the prenatal mutilation became the re-enactment of this mutilation. At this stage, it was clear that the wish to undergo a sex change was related to the excessiveness of Anne as a saturated object of identification. The splitting and projections that characterized Dan's relationship with her positioned her as an object of persecutory wholeness, the identification with which had a psychotic–fetishistic tone. In effect the only way to get rid of this persecutory object was by fusing with it, that is, by becoming it. Yet he experienced the sex change as a cut rather than a caesura: a moment in which he would murder and be murdered, losing both Anne and himself. Dan's desire of gender crossing may be understood as a wish to unite with an object of jouissance—but, no less than that, as a way to annihilate this object by appropriating its identity. The gender dichotomy in this case was psychotically charged by the splitting between Anne's whole face as opposed to his mutilated face, and between her "whole lip" and his "cleft lip", while the gender crossing was aimed at acting out that excess. The psychotherapeutic process can thus be seen as intended to turn "the cleft lip" into a "cleft tongue" (Amir, 2014), that is, to transform the actual cleft into a symbolic one, which can be worked through rather than acted out.

## Discussion

The difference between states of gender crossing that are based on a psychotic organization, like in the case described above, as opposed to transformative gender crossing, is connected to the degree to which the new gender is constituted as a concrete actualization of the phantasm of wholeness. When gender crossing comes to confirm the illusion that it is possible to fill the essential, inherent lack (Lacan, 1958), then, disguised as the realization of subjectivity, it actually undermines this very subjectivity. Oren Gozlan (2015) writes beautifully in this context that "surgery in itself becomes irrelevant to the question of pathology, because what distinguishes an Act from an acting out is not the activity but its ability to be enjoyed as lacking" (p. 54).

"[The] ability to be enjoyed as lacking" requires to preserve the state of lack which enables desire and movement; it means to preserve the unsaturated quality of the concrete act in a way that enables the new state to be constituted and reconstituted in various modes, always absorbing new meanings. Danger appears where gender crossing loses its symbolic quality and becomes a mere concrete act, one which psychotically regenerates the illusion of the primary incestuous union with the original object, as Lacan puts it. What is at stake here is the act itself erasing the experience of lack, so that it becomes an act that nullifies, through the concrete gratification it enables, the very need to create meaning and to enter the symbolic order of language.

This can also be formulated in Bion's (1965) terms as "rigid motion transformations", when a model of relationship is transposed as-is, from one relation to another, without any adjustment. In the context of gender crossing, one can think of a "rigid motion gender crossing" which transfers the typical pattern of saturated gender dichotomy from the old gender to the new gender without enabling a greater freedom vis-a-vis the new gender than vis-a-vis the old one. One can also think of gender crossing as a state of "projective transformations", in which "acidic" contents are projected onto the actual gender, forming a re-lationship of mutual negation with it and paving the way for a gender crossing that negates the negation. Gender crossing can of course be a function of "transformations in hallucinosis", that is, a process whose aim is the evacuation of intolerable contents which can neither be thought of nor represented. Finally, gender crossing may be a function of "transformations in K", that is, an attempt to know the other and otherness, perhaps even take possession of one's otherness.

My assumption is that every gender crossing includes all these transformations in varying degrees of dominance. To return to Dan's case, one can formulate his gender crossing as "rigid motion trans-formations" that transfer the saturated gender dichotomy from the male pole to the female pole without constituting change in Dan's attitude toward gender itself. One can refer to his gender crossing also as "projective transformations", within which acidic persecutory ele-ments were projected upon the actual gender, engaging in a relation-ship in which anything negative was considered a result of this actual male gender, thus "pushing" him to concretely negate his masculinity through its surgical undoing. In addition, one can recognize in Dan's gender crossing elements of "transformations in hallucinosis", that is, the use of the sex change procedures as a form of evacuation and ejection of intolerable elements that cannot be thought of or re-presented. In this type of transformations we can include the psychotic delusion that the mutilation of his face enabled Anne to be born intact, as well as the hallucination that as a result of the surgery he would not only turn into the same sex as Anne, but would actually become Anne. Though one might be misled to perceive Dan's gender crossing as transformations in K, the key element in the wish to "fully know the otherness of Anne" was not really related to the wish to know her, but rather to his unconscious phantasy to take possession of her otherness. All these can explain why in Dan's case gender crossing expressed a psychotic delusion rather than a wish to undergo a true change. In other situations, however, transformations in K could indeed be dominant, and gender crossing be understood as a real striving toward life and liveliness.

## From trans-disciplinarity to inter-disciplinarity

Adrienne Harris (2011) suggests that to work on the phenomenon of transgender subjectivities is to work "trans-disciplinarily" as an enactment of the richness of dimensions and points of view that characterize this phenomenon which obviously "transgresses" the limits of our imagination and thought. One may say that the psychoanalytic work that offers the richest response to the phenomenon of gender crossing is not only "trans-disciplinary" but also "inter-disciplinary": one that focuses not on the actual linear passage from one side to another but rather on the everlasting movement between them, creating thereby a rich caesura in a place that has thus far been formulated only in terms of a cut.

## References

Aharoni, H., & Bergstein, A. (2012). On the Caesura and Some More Caesuras, Foreword to the Hebrew Edition of *Caesura* by Wilfred Bion (trans., Aharoni and Bergstein). Tel-Aviv: Bookworm.

Amir, D. (2012) The Inner Witness. International Journal of Psycho-Analysis, *93*(4), 879–896.

Amir, D. (2014). *Cleft Tongue: The Language of Psychic Structures*. London: Karnac Books.

Amir, D. (2016). *On the Lyricism of the Mind: Psychoanalysis and Literature.* (trans., Mirjam Hadar). London and New York: Routledge.

Bion, W. R. (1962b). *Learning from Experience.* London: Heinemann [Reprinted London: Karnac Books, 1984].

Bion, W. R. (1965). *Transformations.* London: Heinemann.

Bion, W. R. (1967). Catastrophic Change. Unpublished paper.

Bion, W. R. (1970). Container and Contained Transformed. In *Attention and Interpretation.* London: Tavistock [Reprinted London: Karnac books, 1984].

Bion, W. R. (1977). *Two Papers: The Grid and Caesura.* Rio de Janeiro: Imago Editora [Reprinted London: Karnac Books 1989].

Britton, R. (1998). *Belief and Imagination.* New York: Routledge, pp. 120–127.

Gozlan, O. (2015). *Transsexuality and the Art of Transitioning: A Lacanian Approach.* New York: Routledge.

Harris, A. E. (2011). Gender as a Strange Attractor: Discussion of the Transgender Symposium. *Psychoanalytic Dialogues, 21*, 230–238.

Klein, M. (1924). An Obsessional Neurosis in a Six Year Old Girl. In R. Money-Kyrle, B. Joseph, E. O' Shaughnessy, & H. Segal (Eds.). *The Writings of Melanie Klein.* London: The Hogarth Press, Vol. 2, p. 1975.

Lacan, J. ([1958]2007). *Ecrits* (Trans. B. Fink). London: W.W. Norton.

Pesach, H. (2007). *Orlando: A Biography* In V. Woolf (Ed.). Israel: Yediot Books (Hebrew).

Quinodoz, D. (1998). A Fe/Male Transsexual Patient. *International Journal of Psychoanalysis, 79*, 95–111.

Rank, O. (1915). Das Schauspiel im Hamlet. *Imago* 4.

Woolf, V. ([1928]1949). *Orlando: A Biography.* London: The Hogarth Press.

# Chapter 4

# The metaphorical, the metonymical and the psychotic aspects of obsessive symptomatology

The term "obsessional neurosis" (also known as "obsessive-compulsive neurosis", with psychiatrists currently discriminating between obsessive thoughts and compulsive rituals), refers to a class of neuroses identified by Freud, and constituting one of the major frames of reference in psychoanalytic clinical practice:

> In its most typical form of obsessional-neurosis, the psychical conflict is expressed through symptoms which are described as compulsive-obsessive ideas, compulsions towards undesirable acts, struggles against these thoughts and tendencies, rituals etc.—and through a mode of thinking which is characterized in particular by rumination, doubt and scruples, and which leads to inhibitions of both thought and action. (Laplanche & Pontalis, 1973, p. 281)

The present chapter is an attempt to create an integrative formulation of obsessive symptomatology, based on Lacanian and object-relations points of view. I suggest to understand the obsessive symptomatology as manifesting a singular interaction between three aspects which I call "the metaphorical aspect", "the metonymical aspect" and "the psychotic aspect", and which intertwine with a varying degree of dominance. The singular interaction between them crucially affects the capacity for symbolization and reflection, and its implications for analytical work are accordingly far reaching.

Why metaphorical and metonymical?

Metaphor and metonymy are two forms of semantic shift, that is,

DOI: 10.4324/9781003194071-4

two modes of transition from one semantic field to another. Metaphor is the use of a word or expression in a borrowed sense rather than in its simple original meaning, or the use of the characterstics of one concept in order to illuminate another. It is based on analogy, on a relationship of similarity between two semantic fields. The sentence "My lover is a rose" does not imply that the rose itself is the beloved person but that something in the beloved's features resembles those of a rose. Metonymy, by contrast, is a figurative tool that illustrates something by replacing it with something else that is situated close to it in time or space, or that belongs in the same context. The result is not logical in the simple sense and can only be understood through the proximity between the two elements. This is how the expression "the White House" comes to stand for the notion of "the President's spokesperson". As opposed to metaphor, in metonymy there is no transfer of characteristics between the two elements (the President's spokesperson is not meant to share features with the White House). The connection between them is associative only in a way that allows us to perceive the one as representative of the other.

In his article "Two Aspects of Language and Two Types of Linguistic Disturbances" (1956), Roman Jakobson presents metaphor and metonymy as polar opposites rather than parts of the hierarchical order in which they are more commonly seen. He stresses the *similarity* that metaphor installs between its signifiers versus the *contiguity* typical of metonymy. Each of these modes of transposition, he argues, relies on different cognitive skills. While metaphor is based on the cognitive ability to convert, metonymy implies the cognitive ability to connect and contextualize, that is, the ability to create continuity and to identify something as part of—and following from—a context. Jakobson divides the aphasic patients with whom his article is concerned into those who suffer from impaired identification of similarities as opposed to patients whose ability to combine and contextualize is affected. Taking his assumptions into an analytic context, patients with an impaired capacity to identify similarities or to create analogies might be said to suffer from a lack in their symbolic capacity, a condition which may interfere with their capacity to gain from symbolic interventions and interpretations, while patients with an impaired ability to connect and contextualize lack in their capacity to create an emotional continuum that can contain change without turning it into a catastrophic one (Bion, 1970), a condition that might interfere with their very capacity to enter the "analytic play" in the first place.

Lacan's distinction (1958) between metaphor and metonymy diverges from Jakobson's. Though, following the latter, he associates metaphor with the axis of linguistic selection and metonymy with that of combination, metaphor for him acts to constitute meaning while metonymy resists meaning: the metonymic drive is related to the desire to recover the lost Real,[1] while metaphor is associated with the symptom whose creation is a constructive process in which new meaning emerges. Thus, Lacan does not situate metaphor and metonymy as polar opposites—like Jakobson—but rather posits them in a hierarchical order in which patients who (metaphorically) create a symptom are situated higher in terms of their symbolic organization than patients who (metonymically) stick to the attempt to recover the lost pre-linguistic Real.

Following Lacan's and Jakobson's ideas, I would like to discriminate between the metaphorical and the metonymical aspects of obsessive symptomatology, and, furthermore, add a third, "psychotic aspect" to the former two. Simply put, the metaphorical aspect refers to those areas of obsessive symptomatology in which the obsessive thought or the compulsive ritual constitutes a distanced articulation of something the subject is not willing to know. The symptom, in this case, represents both the repressed content and the attempt to repress it. This is how repetitive rescuing thoughts, like repetitive cleaning rituals, can represent an inversion of murderous or "dirty" wishes. The metonymical aspect, on the other hand, refers to those areas of obsessive symptomatology in which the obsessive thought or the compulsive ritual rather than drawing on their specific content, derive their value from the artificial continuum they create through their form of repetition. This compulsive repetition seeks to compensate for a rupture in the sense of self by generating an artificial experience of holding the various parts (of personality) together in a manner that replaces their (im)possible integration. So while the metaphorical solution, which refers mainly to contents or subject-matter, places unacceptable and un-integrated thoughts in a somehow acceptable frame of reference, both allowing and preventing the connection with them through their inversion and displacement—the more primitive metonymical solution has no content-related reference whatsoever but points to a rupture in the experience of self, a rupture which may *cause* the inability to integrate rather than be its consequence.

In contrast with these two aspects, which are amenable and responsive to in-depth interpretation (though differently directed, as I will discuss later), I would like to suggest a third, psychotic aspect. This aspect refers to those areas in which the obsessive symptomatology turns into an addictive object, the powerful union with which acts neither to symbolize repressed contents nor to compensate for the experience of general fragility, but rather to anchor the subject in the territory that precedes language and refuses symbolization. This psychotic aspect is responsible for the addiction to the symptomatology itself. here one can observe a withdrawal to a primitive level of "forclusion",[2] characterized by the refusal of thought, language and otherness, thus constituting an omnipotent psychotic position.

All three aspects (the metaphorical, the metonymical and the psychotic) operate with varying degrees of dominance within every obsessive symptomatology, creating a singular interaction. The question of the type of interaction between the three is crucial, however, since it has important implications for the patient's response to different modes of intervention. While the metaphorical aspect is accessible to in-depth interpretation and stands to gain from bringing to consciousness the repressed contents whose camouflaging it subserves, the interpretive approach appropriate for the metonymical aspect will be experience-near, centering on form rather than content, or on the general rupture in self-contour rather than on the specific contents that leak from it. The psychotic aspect, by contrast, undermines any kind of interpretative work. Analytic work with it must involve presenting concepts of time, space and causal hierarchy that enable separation from the incestuous union with the pre-linguistic object toward the creation of a developed symbolic order.

## The metaphorical aspect

Freud (1926) considered obsessive-compulsive neurosis a repressive process that fails again and again; a defensive move made against unconscious impulses that keep threatening to invade consciousness. In the

"Rat Man" (1909) he claimed that the obsessive-compulsive neurosis is the outcome of oedipal anxiety, causing a regression to anal defenses including reaction-formation, undoing and emotional isolation. In "Inhibitions, Symptoms and Anxiety" (1926), he added a statement about the persecutory and severe nature of the superego when it retreats from a more developed state (characteristic of genital organization) to an archaic one. Hence, Freud regarded obsessive-compulsive neurosis as the individual's defensive regression to the anal-sadistic stage: s/he shuns the dangers involved in the oedipal stage and uses massive defensive maneuvers in order to take control over anal-sadistic impulses (1909, p. 240). This defensive structure struggles against obsessive thoughts while simultaneously giving expression to them (Munich, 1986). Ferenczi (1913) argued that the obsessive person's omnipotent thinking constitutes a regression to the early developmental stage of magical thinking. Abraham (1924) defined obsessive-compulsive neurosis as the libido's anal-sadistic organization, opposing it to melancholy, with the emphasis, in obsession, on controlling and preserving elements, while in melancholy, on destructive ones. This model of obsessive-compulsive neurosis was developed by thinkers such as Nagera (1978), Mallinger (1984) and Salzman (1985). All of these writers thought of it as a collapse of adaptive defenses leading to the activation of secondary means for achieving security, and formulated this collapse in terms of a regression from the oedipal to a pre-oedipal stage (Esman, 2001).

Haft (2005) suggests to combine the classic formulation of obsessive-compulsive neurosis with developments from contemporary, British object-relations theory. She claims that analysis of the transference lays bare the dangerous aggression obsessive patients experience and the terror exercised by the associated destructive impulses. The anal-erotic psychic organization supplies, she suggests, a defense against threats related to the oedipal stage, but puts the very sense of self and object at risk. Primitive fears bring on splitting, idealization, projective-identification and concrete thinking (Steiner, 1987), which are features typical of the anal-sadistic stage (Britton, 1989; Klein, 1945). This results in ongoing damage to the distinct perception of self and object, thus blurring the distinction between internal and external reality. Accompanying this loss of distinction between self and object, there is an extensive use of what Hannah Segal (1957) called *symbol equivalents*: the individual projects his or her destructive impulses onto the world outside where they are concretely experienced as defiling objects, though they are only symbolic re-presentations of the individual's own destructive impulses. This distancing from the true source of danger (i.e., the displacement of threatening in-ternal objects to the external space) serves as a defensive function, yet also generates further anxiety.[3]

These ideas can be understood as referring to what I have above called the metaphorical aspect of obsessive symptomatology, since they treat the obsessive symptomatology as having a status similar to that of a dream object, that is, a symbolic dimension: both the ob-sessive thoughts and the compulsive rituals that come to neutralize them symbolize repressed contents which are projected outward, turning into threatening external objects while actually reflecting the subject's inner world and its destructive impulses. It may be said that the metaphorical aspect of the obsessive symptomatology creates a semantic shift in which the threatening inner objects are placed (ac-tually displaced) in a different territory (an external, concrete one) and inverted (turned into their opposite, for example, turn from dirty thoughts to cleaning rituals). In this move they share the same traits with the original content while disguising it, thereby changing the unbearable object into a bearable one.

## The metonymical aspect

Alongside the rich metaphorical discussion of obsessive symptoma-tology, psychoanalytic thinking has over the years developed a second, "metonymical" (as I call it) model of understanding this phenomenon. Here the focus is not on obsessive symptomatology as bearing on an attempt to avoid contact with anal regression resulting from unresolved oedipal conflicts, but rather on the unconscious attempt to produce—by means of compulsive thoughts and obsessive rituals—an artificial experience of contour and continuity.

In *The Language of Psychoanalysis* Laplanche and Pontalis (1973) write:

A short while after Freud, Janet used the term "psychasthenia" to describe a neurosis close to Freud's obsessional-neurosis, but his conception was centered on a different aetiology: it was a state of deficiency, a weakness of mental synthesis, a psychical asthenia

which Janet held to be fundamental and determined the obsessional struggle itself, whereas for Freud doubts and inhibitions
were the consequence of a conflict which both mobilizes and
blocks the subject's energies. (p. 282)

Janet's understanding of obsessional neurosis focused on the under-
lying mental state of psychasthenia. "Psychasthéniques are characterized by sentiments of psychological incompleteness that are more or
less general, more or less deep, more or less permanent", he wrote
(1908—translated 2010, p. 438). This aetiology may conceal the roots
of the differentiation I am suggesting here between the metaphorical
and the metonymical aspects of obsessive symptomatology. While
Freud ascribed it to unresolved conflicts, Janet ascribed it to mental
weakness. While Freud saw the inability to synthesize (to create a
symbolic integration) as a result, Janet treated it as the primary cause.

As I said before, the metonymical aspect of obsessive symptomatology refers to those areas in which the obsessive thoughts or
compulsive rituals generate an artificial experience of psychic continuity through repetition, compensating for a rupture in the sense of
self. This experience of rupture is not the consequence of an inability
to deal with oedipal conflicts but the very cause of this inability.
O'Connor (2007) suggests, in line with this perception, that the development of obsessive thinking can be considered a product of the
primary environment's defensive function. He proposes that the first
seeds of obsessive thinking can be found in the infant's need to
survive a primary environment which has surrounded it with an
overly protective shell, or, alternatively, which has exposed it to
reality prematurely. In both these extremes, marked by either reduced
or excessive negotiation with reality, the infant fails to internalize a
modulating model that can protect it from its own destructiveness.
Both of these experiences—overexposure and underexposure—are
aspects of the same collapse of the parental object's modulating
ability, leading to the child's failed internalization of a modulating
mechanism. The compulsive rituals therefore constitute an artificial
external modulating object that compensates for the one that did not
generate. For such patients, analytic interpretation may feel like an
intolerable intrusion, which triggers the plethora of obsessive defense
mechanisms with a vengeance. O'Connor's approach obviously ties

in with Winnicott's (1965), concerning the effect of premature impingements and the role of the primary environment in the child's development. But it also refers to later theories concerning the function of the psychic envelope, which simultaneously protects the child from attacks originating in the external world and from impulses generated within.

In 1968, Esther Bick defined the phenomenon of "second skin". In the most primitive phase of infantile development the personality components are felt as having no cohesive power of their own. Much as the different parts of the body require a skin envelope in order to be contained and to form a sense of wholeness and integration, so do the different parts of the personality require a skin-like psychic envelope to contain them and to develop an integrated sense of self. When the primary object fulfills the function of a skin container this function is internalized, enabling the infant in due time to generate an inner container of its own. But in the absence of this experience the infant is left with an experience of non-containment. In order not to suffer the unbearable sense of un-integration, the psyche generates an artificial envelope that is felt to hold the internal parts together. The second skin has various manifestations, both physical and mental: muscular rigidity, movement rituals, sticking to certain items of clothing, compulsive thinking, or even maintaining a rigid routine—all these may function as a second skin. Following Bick's ideas, Ogden (1989) proposed an autistic-contiguous position as a way of conceptualizing a psychological organization that is more primitive than the paranoid-schizoid position. The autistic-contiguous mode is a sensory-dominated, pre-symbolic mode of experience. Anxiety in this mode consists of an unspeakable terror of the dissolution of boundedness, resulting in feelings of leaking, falling forever or dissolving into endless, shapeless space. Patients' attempt in this position to create a sense of boundedness can take many forms of repetitive self-soothing actions. Ogden further suggests that compulsive masturbation, as well as compulsive procrastination, may also be understood as two forms of an attempt to create a sensory boundedness. Compulsive masturbation keeps the body in a state of permanent arousal which serves as a contour, holding the person's various parts together. Compulsive procrastination achieves the same target in a different way: the existence of a deadline is a source of constant pressure, supplying a sense of boundary, albeit a threatening and disturbing one. Release, in both cases, is only momentary. Orgasm, for masturbators, and fulfilling a task, in the case of procrastinators, actually heighten the level of anxiety effacing the sensory boundary and the sense of demarcation it produces. Ogden argues that obsessive defenses are always related to the effort to sensorially fill in holes in the experience of the self, holes through which the subject fears his or her mental and bodily contents may seep out. Compulsive symptoms, he further claims, do not originate in unresolved sexual conflicts but rather in the psyche's unstinting effort to artificially produce a sense of boundedness.

Ogden's and Bick's approaches pinpoint what I call the metonymical aspect of obsessive symptomatology. When this metonymical aspect is dominant, the subject of analytical work is the experience of leakage and absence of contours, rather than the specific unconscious conflicts hidden under this obsessive symptomatology or leaking through it; not repressed sexuality or aggression, shame or guilt, but rather a deep rupture in the continuous experience of the self which the obsessive repetition comes to repair.

Hinshelwood (1997) writes:

> Skin sensation is quickly joined by other perceptions. The sensations from various other organs are experienced in the same way. The mouth, the eyes, the hands are all used similarly at first; each hole is closed by some object that completes the sense of boundary—the nipple in the mouth, a point of light for the eyes, a hard object for the hand, etc. They represent the same two possibilities—open and leaking, or closed and filled by an object. Attention to that object "fills" a catastrophic hole in the boundary. (p. 309)

The metonymical aspect is in charge of those areas in the obsessive symptomatology in which the symptomatology itself serves as the object that fills "the catastrophic hole in the boundary" Hinshelwood mentions. Compensating for the inability to integrate the various parts of the personality, the obsessive mechanisms create an artificial experience whereby the various parts are mechanically and passively held together (contrary to the active containing of the metaphoric aspect) through the repetitive rituals and thoughts, creating thereby a hard carapace which seemingly protects the inner core while actually serving to replace it. Returning to Janet's understanding of obsessional neurosis as characterized by "sentiments of psychological incompleteness", the metonymical aspect refers to those areas of obsessive symptomatology that are in charge of the need to maintain the obsessive ritual not as a defense against unbearable conflict (which assumes a neurotic organization) but as a means to keep one's weak, underdeveloped self together in one piece.

## The psychotic aspect

The psychotic aspect of obsessive symptomatology, as I suggest defining it, refers to those areas of the obsessive symptomatology where the symptomatology itself turns into an addictive object, one with whom the primary union acts to anchor the subject in the territory of the Real. Through the obsessive thoughts and the compulsive rituals this aspect preserves a magical union with the primary maternal object, thus neutralizing the symbolic order along with the subject qua subject within language. In order to describe how this malignant transformation takes place, I would like to introduce some of Lacan's ideas concerning psychotic thinking, using them to explain the essence of the psychotic aspect of obsessive symptomatology as well as the unique analytic work it requires.

Subjectivity begins with the process of signification. What exists before language is a state of what we might call pure presence, in which the pre-linguistic infant experiences a timeless, disjoint sense of self. In this state of formlessness, the infant, unable to distinguish between self and other, merges with its environment and particularly with its mother (Clowes, 2003). Lacan (1977) calls this a-temporality the "here and now". With the acquisition of language, this state of pure presence comes to an end all at once. Along with the process of signification comes subjectivity, through the construction of a series of discrete representations and identifications that bring the child into temporality, sociality and the symbolic order. There is, however, always a surplus that stays outside these representations. Lost in the process of symbolization, this surplus stays outside the order of language and becomes the object of desire (*object a*). According to Lacan, language, form and identity all arise from the opposite principle of the void. Lacan (1992) refers to this void at the center of language as "das Ding", the absent "thing" to which all signifiers refer but with which they cannot coincide. Psychic motion is always directed toward this object of desire, and it is through this motion that the subject is constituted qua living subject. One can imagine this core object of desire as the place where, if one could only reach it, one would experience pure, unmediated satisfaction. For subjects, who are by definition situated within language, though, it is impossible to revert either to *das Ding* or to the primitive, undifferentiated environment of the pre-linguistic "here and now" (Clowes, 2003). Thus, in contrast with the concept of the object as satisfactory, Lacan introduces the absent object as constitutive to the emergence of the subject in the first place. No psychic motion will be possible without the experience of lack.

Returning to the psychotic aspect of obsessive symptomatology, I would like to suggest that this psychotic aspect refers exactly to those areas in which the obsessive symptomatology creates, as a result of its intensity and its overpowering pervasiveness, an illusion of reverting to the pre-linguistic "here and now" and to the merger with the pre-linguistic mother. Lacan (1958) writes that "the symbol first manifests itself as the killing of the thing, and this death results in the endless perpetuation of the subject's desire" (p. 262). In his terms, the psychotic aspect might be said to be in charge of the areas in which the obsessive symptomatology does not "kill the thing" by constituting a symbol that comes to replace it, but rather erases the basic experience of lack (and along with it the basic experience of desire) which is crucial for subjectivity to break through and enter symbolization and language. These are the areas in which the obsessive symptomatology creates a unique masochistic fulfillment of the regressive urge to unite with the breast and the mother, generating a phantasm of wholeness which paradoxically combines pain with jouissance.

There is a crucial difference between the metaphorical and the psychotic aspects of obsessive symptomatology: while the former, which creates the symptom as a defense against the temptation to dwell in the phantasmatic jouissance, seeks to preserve both the experience of lack and the need to create meaning, the latter, psychotic aspect appears where the symptom collapses as such, namely, when it turns from being what signifies the hole, into "the thing" that fills in that hole. In addition to the above, it is important to discriminate the metonymical aspect from the psychotic: while the former preserves subjectivity through an ongoing contact with the experience of rupture, using obsessive symptomatology as a means to withstand it—the latter actually attacks the very experience of rupture, using the obsessive symptomatology to create an illusory wholeness in which there are neither needs nor the urge to fulfill them.

Since we are dealing here with a hierarchy of symbolization, the metonymic aspect can be conceived of as situated before the psychotic collapse takes over: the use of the obsessive symptomatology to heal ruptures in the sense of self can be understood as a defense against the complete collapse of subjectivity through the use of the obsessive symptomatology as an object of merger.

These three aspects (the metaphoric, metonymic and psychotic) can also be put in terms of Bion's (1970) three types of interaction, here between subject and symptomatology: the metaphoric aspect of obsessive symptomatology may be understood as the aspect which is in charge of a symbiotic interaction, in which the symptom contains the hidden contents in a way that both communicates them and allows them to painfully absorb meaning through symbolic interpretation. The metonymic aspect can be seen as the aspect in charge of a commensal interaction, characterized by mutual coexistence of subject and symptomatology, in a kind of status quo which neither leads to significant development nor causes psychotic collapse. Finally, the psychotic aspect can be thought of as enacting a parasitic interaction in which the symptomatology destroys the subject who malignantly and magically clings to it. According to Bion, the psychotic personality, full of envy and hatred of dependence, makes destructive attacks on the part of the mental apparatus that registers sense impressions. As a result of this massive use of fragmentation and projection, omnipotence and omniscience substitute for thinking (Lucas, 1992, p. 73). What Lacan adds to Bion's theory on psychosis is the special focus on the masochistic jouissance, which may be used to explain both the subject's powerful clinging to the painful obsessive symptomatology as well as the latter's undermining of subjectivity not merely through the annihilation of thinking but also through the erasure of the basic experience of lack which elicits the urge to create meaning. As the following detailed clinical illustration demonstrates, the combination of pain and jouissance is crucial to understanding the psychotic aspect of obsessive symptomatology.

Although the three aspects of obsessive symptomatology were described in three separate sections so far, this chapter's aim is not to deal with them separately but to portray the complex collage they create, contributing the varying components of fundamentally the same phenomenon. The detailed clinical illustration below is an attempt to capture these three aspects at work and analyze their interaction in the obsessive symptomatology of a young woman.

## Clinical illustration

Ophelia, a woman in her mid-thirties, turns to analysis due to a severe outbreak of intrusive, violent thoughts following the birth of her first child. She has suffered from such thoughts since early adolescence but this current round is unbearable. She receives medication but feels that it is not enough. In our first meeting she presents me with an extremely difficult family story. She is the youngest daughter of a rather weak (but loving) father and an extremely violent mother who was wont to shift between excessive worry for her children and abuse, especially whenever they tried to assert their independent will. The abuse included hitting them, locking them out of the house in the middle of the night, forcing them to eat food they had spat out, curses and humiliations, also in the presence of others.

Ophelia suffers from intrusive thoughts that invade her many times daily. The thoughts concern her son whom she imagines being taken captive, undergoing severe torture. The thoughts (and the flickering images that come along with them) arouse great anxiety, which she soothes by means of compulsive counting rituals in which she counts cars, people and her own acts (steps, eye blinks, breaths). Other times are dominated by rituals that involve circular movements. These rituals have no thoughts attached to them, but rather respond to an amorphous need that arises in waves. She drives in circles around the city's squares, runs in circles around her house, circles the yard of the school she attended as a child, walking heel-to-toe. The circular movement itself, she says, relaxes her. There are moments, though, when the "thing" (this is the word she uses) becomes so powerful that she no longer has thoughts, and a powerful buzz in her head takes over, a buzz that doesn't allow any thoughts, neither intrusive nor otherwise. As analysis progressed, what occurred to me was that those "buzz" moments were not just moments of attack on thinking but also constituted a regressive experience of Fusion and wholeness. They had, in Ophelia's own words (always in retrospect, though), a kind of anestheticizing quality. While lingering in them, she wanted nothing more, nothing less. In such a state she had no feelings of hate, no guilt, no bouts of longing. She felt no pressure to take care of anything: not her child, not her marriage, not her professional career. All she wanted was to be allowed to dwell in this "thing" that both filled and wrapped her at the same time. It was a kind of torturing pleasure, addictive not in spite of the pain but rather because of it.

Ophelia presented, it may be said, a complex collage of the three aspects of obsessive symptomatology: the metaphorical aspect was the one in charge of the incessant, intrusive thoughts and images. This aspect generated her phenomenological distress and probably also motivated her seeking for help. The metonymical aspect, which expressed itself in the circling and some of the counting rituals, became dominant when Ophelia's general sense of self became too fragile. The metonymic rituals were not a reaction to intrusive contents but rather to a somewhat undifferentiated and general weakness. The circling was experienced not as violent inner coercion but rather as calming actions which eventually enabled her to go back to her daily routine and function in it, at least partially. The psychotic aspect, on the other hand, had an opposite effect: it did not enable her to function; actually it got in the way of functioning. When this aspect took the upper hand Ophelia dwelled, totally immersed, in a place she experienced as a hermetic womb and which she had no desire to leave. The "buzz", as she described it, acted as a mechanical noise-blurring which masked all other external and internal noises. What accompanied it was not plain jouissance, but one with a masochistic tone. It seemed that this masochistic jouissance repeated the quality of the incestuous union with her mother, one which she always experienced as painful and satisfying much to the same extent.

Ophelia's intrusive thoughts began during her compulsory army service. One day she took home a classified video-cassette by mistake. When she discovered what had happened, she was flooded by anxiety and decided, on her mother's advice, to burn it in the back yard.

But the incident did not stop troubling her. She started to suffer from the intrusive thought that the burnt remains had fallen into the enemy's hands and that if a soldier were to be attacked it would be her fault. This thought had gone on tormenting her for years, changing shape from time to time. Its current version, though, was the most difficult of all: ever since her son was born she couldn't help imagining him being kidnapped and tortured by terrorists. When she turned to analysis, the severity and flooding were so powerful that she could hardly function. It was also taking its toll on her marital life.

We began a four times a week analysis. At times, when the anxiety attacks intensified and she was unable to contain them, she asked for a fifth meeting. It wasn't always possible, and with time I understood that it wasn't necessarily right either. The importance of a fixed setting crystallized as analysis proceeded, and I evolved a sense of the role it fulfilled in Ophelia's experience of boundedness. At first she found it very difficult to lie on the couch, fearing to lose eye contact with me and remain on her own. There were sessions in which she abruptly sat up on the couch and proclaimed that she must see if I was still there. Sometimes she remained seated throughout the entire session. In most cases, however, a meaningful interpretation helped her lie down again. A meaningful interpretation was one that was attuned to the dominant aspect of her symptomatology. When the dominant aspect was metonymical, I could tell her, for example, that my silences were like holes through which she was being dropped again and again, and that she needed to fix those holes by the meeting of her eyes with mine. On the other hand, when the dominant aspect was metaphorical, she might sit up because she felt that she was collapsing under the intensity of her aggressive projections on me, and had to assure that I myself was not collapsing as well. When this was the situation, only interpretations that related to her phantasies of destroying me (i.e., metaphorical interpretations, ones that referred to her repressed, displaced wishes) could calm her down. When, however, the dominant aspect was psychotic, there was no point at all in interpreting her sitting up, and the only possibility was to contain her restlessness without forcing any meaning upon it. During one of those moments she began shifting restlessly on the couch, creating something that looked like a compulsive continuum—turning to the right and then to the left in an apparently regular pattern. She seemed to be cradling herself, and was also completely withdrawn (this "hermetic" state, somehow combining pleasure with suffering, signaled the shift to the psychotic aspect). Hush ..., I said to her very quietly, almost in a whisper. Hush. What was going on in my mind when this happened? I sensed she needed a sign I was still there, yet without interrupting her movements. "Hush" was my way to signal my presence without forcing symbolic meaning (through using words) on her fragility. She slowly relaxed after three or four minutes and stopped moving. Only then was it possible to tell her something about her withdrawn restlessness, and about my feeling that she wanted me to call her back yet at the same time leave her untouched.

In effect, I could map every analytical session in terms of the movement between these three aspects. Each time my interpretation didn't coincide with the dominant aspect, Ophelia somehow rejected or ignored it, although she wasn't conscious of it. Thus, for instance, if I was about to interpret her sitting on the couch as an attempt to deal with the intensity of her aggressiveness, while what she was experiencing was a lack of outline, my interpretation (experienced as violent and rude) seemed to have expanded the holes in her experience of self (as well as in the continuity of our relationship), that is, the very holes through which she felt she was being dropped. On the other hand, if I were to interpret her need for contour while she was busy destroying me in her phantasies, I might strengthen her feeling that she was really destroying me, or at least my analytical capacities, leading me astray so that I wouldn't see her for what she was.

In the course of the second year of analysis, Ophelia entered her second pregnancy and gave birth to a baby girl. Her anxiety around the birth of her daughter reached unprecedented peaks. Around this period thoughts about being hospitalized began to flood her. Her fantasy was not about a psychiatric hospitalization, but rather about a medical situation that would demand 24 hours care, far away from home. When I tried to explore this fantasy, Ophelia told me that at the age of four she had had a strep throat, running a high temperature. She remembers how her mother looked after her devotedly, as she always did when Ophelia was ill, but as her temperature rose, her mother grew more and more anxious until she started shaking Ophelia and shouting: "Make up your mind! *You* say if you want to go to the hospital! *You* decide, I can't decide on my own!" Perhaps out of fear, perhaps understanding that her mother was no longer able to look after her, Ophelia asked to be taken to the hospital.

She remembers how calm she grew when the doctors took over, and her sense of security and serenity when her mother left her there and went home. Ophelia is a great hospital aficionado as a grown-up, too: she takes advantage of any opportunity to visit ER and rest there. She tells me that the intrusive thoughts always stop when she gets there, as though she feels the healthiest when she is hospitalized. I would like to present now a clinical vignette that relates to the subject of hospitalization, in order to illustrate the way in which the different aspects of Ophelia's symptomatology interweave:

*Ophelia:* I don't think you have any idea what's running through my mind when I imagine my son growing up. I imagine him walking in the street, kind of happy, and then all sorts of invasions of horrible images: he's kidnapped, tied up to a chair with iron chains, his fingernails and toenails torn out one by one so that he tells them secrets he doesn't even know (She bitterly weeps). It's all because of me, you understand? Because of that video-cassette I accidentally stole. Because of me he will pay.

*Analyst:* Again and again, you describe a horrifying, nightmarish scene, in which you and your son are helpless against outside aggressors. Perhaps it's even more frightening to think that all the parts of this scene actually belong to you. That there is a part in you that wants to save your son but also a part that can have difficult emotions toward him, a part that wants to hurt him and take vengeance against him, maybe even because of the heartache and worry he causes you by his very being.

*Ophelia:* But I want to save him all the time, if I would have wanted something bad to happen to him I wouldn't be so tormented by these visions, don't you think? And why would I even want something bad to happen to him?

*Analyst:* I think your attitude toward him is complex, and within it all sorts of forces might be at play, just like with your mother's attitude toward you, where forces of love and hate operated in a way that made it impossible to differentiate them at times. Maybe you simultaneously want to prevent anything from happening to him but also struggle with the thought that if only he were never born, you wouldn't suffer so deeply.

*Ophelia*
*(after a silence):* I'll tell you something I've never told anyone in my life. I hope I won't regret saying it to you now. Sometimes, when I perform my oath whispers (she is referring to a form of prayers for her son's wellbeing which she whispers daily in a fixed order), some "opposing whispers" sneak in. Do you understand what an "opposing whisper" is?

*Analyst:* Tell me about it.

*Ophelia:* For instance, yesterday, when I said the part of "and may you never be left alone", an opposite sentence suddenly sneaked in, and I found myself saying "If only you were left alone". I quickly erased it and said the correct sentence over and over again so that the opposing one disappeared. But now, when you said what you said, I couldn't help thinking of it. Sometimes I feel that I'm really contaminating him with my thoughts. Sometimes I think that if I stay by his side he'll be infected by my disease. That's why I didn't breastfeed him, you understand? I was afraid I might infect him through my milk.

*Analyst:* It frightens you so much to think that you are capable of harming him, or of feeling such difficult emotions toward him, that anything else is preferable: even staging an entire, horrifying inner scene in which others torture him, provided that you remain the savior and not the aggressor. But you're actually telling me more than that. You're telling me that as long as you don't confront your real emotions you can release neither yourself nor him from the scene of torture.

Following this significant exchange a long silence prevailed. Then Ophelia said she would like to go straight to the hospital and be hospitalized since these thoughts were unbearable for her. I told her that it seemed that hospitalization was the only way to take a break from the monstrous maternal part that persecuted her from within, threatening to drive her mad. Hospital symbolized for her a zone of sanity, a space where there was a clear law, a transparent hierarchy and an unambiguous concept of who takes care of whom, and within which she was confident that taking care of her meant keeping her alive and not putting her to death.

With hindsight, I could see the wish to be hospitalized as constituting an area of condensation generated by the three aspects of Ophelia's symptomatology: in terms of the metaphorical aspect, as exemplified by the vignette above, the wish to be hospitalized may be understood as the wish to escape from her monstrous internal contents. In terms of the metonymical aspect, the wish to be hospitalized may be understood as the wish to fix, through ongoing and close medical attention, the holes in her experience of self, holes that can also be understood in terms of the difficulty of integrating the good and the bad, the deadening and the vitalizing parts of her own internal objects. In terms of the psychotic aspect, the wish to be hospitalized could be seen as an expression of Ophelia's wish not to think, not to dream, not to be; the wish to be completely merged with her addicting pain; the wish to anesthetize her thinking apparatus and in that way neutralize not merely the specific thoughts that she couldn't bear thinking, but also the thinking subject that she couldn't bear to be.[4]

In the months preceding the birth of her second child, Ophelia repeatedly announced that she did not intend to take maternity leave. She planned to leave the baby with a caretaker and return to work a few days after delivery. She didn't want to nurse the baby and had no interest whatsoever in mothering as long as the baby was too young to communicate. She was struggling with feelings of alienation and indifference, and could only think of the injustice the birth of her daughter would do to her eldest son. When she finally had the baby, however, something changed. She started breastfeeding, reporting anxiety but also a sense of closeness to the infant, and she even changed the baby's original name to one that had some connection to her own name. A moment of relief was registered, immediately upon which her intrusive thoughts took on a new shape: she said that if it were up to her, it would have been better if her son had never been born and she were solely the mother of her daughter, whom she experienced as less needy and less exposed to danger. Subsequently she said that it wasn't just that she wished he had never been born, but that she would like him to die: only his death could put an end to her torturous concern for his being. Though she reported that her relationship with her daughter was good and intimate, wholly unlike the fraught relations with her son, she started talking about the need to stop breastfeeding so that "the baby will be accessible to all". I felt (and interpreted) that these words concealed a wish for this baby, too, to be taken away from her. This interpretation related to the metaphoric aspect of her illness, trying to help her understand her decision to stop breastfeeding the baby as another sign of her aggressive wishes which she was simultaneously acting out as well as trying to protect her baby from. This interpretation led her to bring the baby along with her to some of our meetings. Watching her with her little baby-girl was a complex and difficult experience. She sat on the armchair in front of me, holding the sleeping baby in her arms, sometimes patting her small body as if it were her own thigh. Her manner of holding the baby resembled the way one would hold an object or a doll. Leaning forward to take her glasses out of her bag she squashed the infant's body several times; on another occasion she lifted and put the child down without relating to its facial expression, her own face staying expressionless, too. I sensed that her mothering was full of denied hatred, violence, sadism (she called her daughter "entrecote", for instance, or "a cut of meat"). She often said, explicitly, regarding her relationship with her daughter: "It's a crazy (very intense, that is) connection". With time I learned how ambiguous this expression was. The madness was there, indeed, in full force.

With hindsight I understood that sitting face to face with me while holding the baby was also an unconscious enactment of her inner conflicts. Perhaps she wished to check how I withstood her aggression toward the baby. If I withstood her aggression, perhaps she could withstand it too. Perhaps she wished to check how I dealt with my own counter-transference aggression. If I were to offer her a modeling of coping with my aggression, perhaps she would believe that

I could also help her cope with her own. It is also possible, though, to understand her choice to bring the baby along as an expression of the metonymical aspect of her illness. The bigger her hatred grew—the less contained she felt. It is possible that she needed, especially at that time, my continuous gaze as well as my continuous holding as a re-assurance that she had my permission to go on being.

As analysis progressed it became clear that Ophelia's intrusive thoughts were far from coincidental. They counteracted every ex-pression of tenderness, love or yearning, as though attacking the slightest hint of her goodness. She was afraid to feel love for anyone because bad thoughts immediately stirred. She was afraid to smile or even be momentarily happy because she immediately found herself under attack. In analysis the image of a floodgate emerged, behind which tenderness and violence were locked together. Each time a crack opened and something soft filtered through, along, too, came in the most violent devils. Because of the pathological enmeshment of love and hate which characterized Ophelia's internalized objects she was unable not only to integrate them but also to differentiate them. Thus, she experienced love itself as an annihilating power. This pattern was enacted in the analytic relationship too: she made every possible effort to gain my love but was mortified whenever I ex-pressed any affection or compassion. While she was insulted when confronted by a boundary, she was also frightened when she sus-pected an absence of boundaries. When I was, in her own words, "being good to her" she became contemptuous, but whenever she experienced me as remote she became terrified. She was in a trap, hovering between her huge yearning for contact and the feeling that contact was a matter of death, not life.

## Discussion

Ophelia's severe symptomatology was a combination of all three aspects. There was no question about the symbolic (metaphoric) nature of her intrusive thoughts which split off her destructive wishes and the repressed sadism toward her children. The forbidden content underwent con-densation and displacement, diverting her aggression toward her children to foreign territories, shifting the execution scene from home to Syrian captivity. The repetitive counting rituals that had a clear undoing function were, at least partially, metaphorical too: these activities actually represented an attempt to "settle accounts", or—alternatively—"to account for her bad thoughts". But besides their metaphorical quality those counting rituals also had a clear metonymical aspect, where they sought to compensate for Ophelia's lack of inner continuity, maybe even fighting possible psychotic fragmentation by maintaining mechanical order and hierarchy through counting. Even if the metaphorical aspect allowed for some measure of interpretive analytical work, sharp shifts from the dominance of this aspect to the dominance of the metonymical and the psychotic aspects could be clearly observed. The metonymical aspect was reflected mostly in her repetitive circling, whose soothing effect must have been related to the restoring of cyclic continuity. The repetitive circling can clearly be seen as an act aimed to heal ruptures in Ophelia's self-experience and to compensate for the missing psychic envelope by means of creating a sort of "second skin" (Bick, 1968). She said, in this context, that circling felt like enveloping, every circle creating another layer of protective matter. Swings to the dominance of the psychotic aspect were most manifest when her thoughts lost their shape and turned into what she called a "buzz" in her head. Unlike the intrusive thoughts, this buzz constituted an attack on the ability to have any thought at all, an attack on the entire thinking apparatus. Interestingly enough, even when the metaphorical rather than the psychotic aspect was in ascendancy, there were still indications of psychotic attacks on thinking and symbolization which were expressed, for instance, in Ophelia's lack of adequate concepts of space and time, cause and effect. This was, for instance, why she did not think of the incident with the classified video-cassette as an event that belonged in the past, but rather as something ongoing, for which even 20 years later her son might still have to pay the price. This is also why Ophelia couldn't distinguish inside from outside: her inner objects kept turning into persecutory external ones. Lastly, this was why real external objects lost their specificity and contours as they underwent ever increasing generalizations: the soldier, for instance, who was in danger of being kidnapped as a result of the incident with the classified video-cassette 20 years ago, blended with the figure of her son who now became the likely present object of kidnap. Lacking the capacity for creating spatial, temporal or causal differentiations, she could tolerate no contact with her aggression since such contact, once made, was experienced as never ending.

As I said above, the three aspects do not exist separately but create a specific dynamic interaction. This is why even when the content and form of Ophelia's intrusive thoughts were metaphoric, they were still saturated with a psychotic quality that undermined their symbolic level. In the ongoing circular experience produced by the psychotic aspect of Ophelia's symptomatology, movement of thought became horizontal. While intrusive thinking spread, taking in more and more objects, it resisted any kind of "crossing" with insight, or with a more objective type of thinking. Whereas the metaphorical aspect used the obsessive rituals to somehow distribute the indistinct, generalized lump of evil—which had a compartmentalizing function, putting the infinite scene on a time line or even on an apparently causal continuum—the psychotic aspect caused the rituals—even when they still maintained their formal metaphoric outline—to lose their compartmentalizing function, issuing in a meaningless, everlasting sequence.

There were other expressions of psychotic circular logic that infiltrated the metaphorical sequences, too: the confusion, for instance, between being herself the baby whom her mother hurt, and her being the mother who might hurt her own babies. Furthermore, the experience of herself as hurting her son was actually an inversion of her sense of being swallowed, raped and taken over by him. Lastly, this experience of the child dominating her was also an inversion of her own infantile experience of her mother as raping and devouring her. In this circular psychotic symmetry (Matte-Blanco, 1975, 1988), hence, her son became her mother whom she attacked in order to prevent him from attacking her. Victim and victimizer traded places incessantly.

The hospital episode was another example of this circularity. In this scene the child was forced by the mother to take the latter's role, having to make up her mind about whether or not to be hospitalized. The calming effect of the hospital therefore related to the return of hierarchy. Where it was clear that the doctors were to take responsibility and that the child was the one being cared for, some degree of order was restored. This is why, also in her adult life, whenever she re-entered the circularity of intrusive thinking, her first intuition was to get herself hospitalized. Such moments occurred for instance whenever she threw up (which was always attended by huge anxiety), fearing she might drown in her own vomit. Here, too, inside and outside mingled; the body's inside threatened to devour its outside, so that she needed to bring herself to a place where there was a soothing hierarchy, where order reigned and inside and outside were put back into their respective places.

In a recurrent dream Ophelia finds herself jailed in her parents' house, unable to get out. She keeps asking "Where are my children? Where is my husband?" In fact she is stuck in an a-temporal space that constantly reruns the traumatic Real, with no possibility to mourn, to separate, to create an inner representation or to constitute subjectivity.

Fink (1989) discusses the importance of introducing concepts of time and space (these come under the metaphorical aspect) where they don't exist. I consider Ophelia's analysis one whose deep significance consisted in restoring hierarchy and bringing in "symmetry breaking" elements which released her from the psychotic domain of symmetrical circular thinking (Matte-Blanco, 1975, 1988).

One day she arrived earlier than expected and I asked her to wait in my waiting room. Her reaction was extreme. She stamped her feet, smashed her glasses, stayed silent throughout the entire session and eventually said she could not talk to me because I obviously preferred my other patients over her (I was in a session with another patient when she arrived). For the duration of three or four meetings she remained obsessively preoccupied with this issue but eventually admitted that there had been something soothing in the fact that I did not go along with her and apologized. One might of course consider her reaction as a narcissistic rage or a borderline reaction to being faced with a boundary. I would rather think of it in terms of introducing a temporal object into the a-temporality characterizing the territory marked by the psychotic aspect of her symptomatology. The fact that I did not ignore time as she did, inserting, rather, concepts of time into the domain of symmetrical logic (thereby clarifying that my time was not her time), as well as concepts of space (the space of my consulting room is sometimes occupied by someone else) and of hierarchy (I was the one who set the rules, not she)—all this eventually soothed her. Asserting these symmetry breaking and generalization breaking parameters was extremely valuable to the therapeutic process. Introducing hierarchic elements in the form of a role division (I set the rules), time division and time order (early or late), a spatial division (inside and outside, also in the sense of in the consulting room or outside it; within the time frame and outside it) transformed the shapeless lump of hatred and anxiety, boundless and indistinct, into something that could be divided and measured, and therefore create a meaningful scene.

Having come to understand the relations and interactions between the three aspects of Ophelia's symptomatology, my analytic interventions were of three kinds (sometimes, when I perceived a mixture of a metaphoric or metonymic quality with a psychotic one, I obviously sought to respond to that mixture by identifying the most dominant aspect and relate to it):

a.  Interventions aimed at the metaphorical aspect: these interventions touched upon the violent wishes and thoughts she displaced onto external objects which then became persecutory. Thus, the focus of interpretation was on her unconscious wishes and thoughts.
b.  Interventions addressing the metonymical aspect: these interventions were experience-near, touching upon the ritual itself (in terms of its form and not its content) as having an enveloping and healing quality. This aimed to enable her to be less exposed and fragile and more capable of dealing with external and internal reality.
c.  Interventions addressing the psychotic aspect: these interventions were possible only in retrospect. Within Ophelia's psychotic "buzz" there was neither place nor need for interpretation, nor was there a container that might hold any link. In retrospect, however, it was possible to touch on what I perceived as the psychotic circular aspect of her obsessive rituals and repetitive thoughts, as creating a kind of hermetic wholeness, both painful and satisfying, which silenced the unbearable external and internal noises (thoughts, emotions, needs), even at the cost of thinking and feeling, even at the cost of being.

The great difficulty in working analytically with obsessive symptomatology may be connected to the fact that analytical interpretations mostly refer to the metaphorical and the metonymical aspects and are less attentive to the psychotic aspect of this phenomenon. Furthermore, since in some cases the psychotic aspect may be not asymbolic (as in complete psychosis) but rather pseudo-symbolic, it is of particular importance to identify it, mainly because when it is not identified the analytical interpretations, focusing on the obsessive "pseudo-thoughts", may remain detached or become malignant and addictive objects in themselves. However, as soon as it is acknowledged and the symmetrical circular logic in which it operates is taken into account, analysis may focus on introducing symmetry breaking means, ones that can constitute, step by step, a hierarchy of space, time and causality, with the aim of boosting a thinking apparatus that may contain metaphoric interpretations later on. Mapping the unique interaction between these three aspects of obsessive symptomatology and adapting the interpretative work to that interaction may, therefore, create a richer matrix for development as well as for change.

## Notes

1 Lacan's concept of the Real refers to what is outside language and resists symbolization.
2 In "A question prior to any possible treatment of psychosis" (1958) Lacan writes about the notion of "forclusion" in the context of psychosis. Repression and forclusion differ in that while the first aims to remove a thought or an image from consciousness, the latter removes it from the unconscious. In other words, while forclusion casts the materials out of the unconscious, repression strives to fix them there. While repression is part of normal psychic functioning—though under certain conditions it has neurotic outcomes that impair functioning—forclusion consists of a violent rejection of psychic reality and its implications are catastrophic. It leads to psychosis rather than neurosis.
3 McDougall (1999, p. 62) mentions in this context a patient who presented an ideal figure: saintly, maternal, someone who treated all of humanity with generosity and love. This figure, however, concealed another, very different one: diabolical, wild and full of hate toward children. The patient used complicated compulsive rituals in order to keep control of this hidden figure. McDougall presents an episode in which the patient complimented her on the flowers on her table and then fell silent. When McDougall asked her to continue, she said that it suddenly occurred to her that McDougall may have been too old to have children and that's why she grew flowers instead. McDougall draws attention to the aggression concealed by the compliment, the hatred behind the manifest admiration.
4 As analysis progressed, though, and in a way that I understand as a significant achievement, the wish to be hospitalized changed from being the wish to anesthetize her thinking to being an expression of the wish to gain back the laws of reality and thinking: to reconstruct a space in which hierarchies and differentiations were maintained.

# References

Abraham, K. (1924). A Short Study of the Development of the Libido in the light of Mental Disorders. I. Melancholia and Obsessional Neurosis. *Selected Papers*. New York: Basic Books, pp. 422–433, 1953.

Bick, E. (1968). The Experience of the Skin in Early Object-Relations. *International Journal of Psycho-Analysis*, 49, 484–486.

Bion, W. R. (1957). Differentiation of the Psychotic from the Non-Psychotic Personalities. *Second Thoughts*. London: Heinemann; New York: Aronson, 1967.

Bion, W. R. (1970). *Attention and Interpretation*. London: Tavistock [Reprinted London: Karnac Books, 1984].

Bion, W. R. (1967). Catastrophic Change. Unpublished paper.

Britton, R. (1989). The Missing Link: Parental Sexuality in the Oedipus Complex. In J. Steiner (Ed.). *The Oedipus Complex Today: Clinical Implications*. London: Karnac Books.

Clowes, E. K. (2003). Regressive Nostalgia in Teshigahara's Woman in the Dunes. *Fort Da*, 9, 70–86.

Esman, A. H. (2001). Obsessive-Compulsive Disorder: Current Views. *Psychoanalytic Inquiry*, 21, 145–156.

Ferenczi, S. (1913), Stages in the Development of the Sense of Reality. *Sex in Psychoanalysis*. New York: Basic Books, pp. 213–239, 1950.

Fink, K. (1989). From Symmetry to Asymmetry. *International Journal of Psycho-Analysis*, 70, 481–489.

Freud, S. (1909). Notes Upon a Case of Obsessional Neurosis. *Standard Edition*. London: Hogarth Press, Vol. 10, pp. 155–318, 1955.

Freud, S. (1926). Inhibitions, Symptoms and Anxiety. *Standard Edition*. London: Hogarth Press, Vol. 20, pp. 87–175. 1959.

Haft, J. (2005). On My Way Here, I Passed a Man with a Scab. *Psychoanalytic Quarterly*, 74, 1101–1126.

Hinshelwood, R. D. (1997). Catastrophe, Objects and Representation: Three Levels of Interpretation. *British Journal of Psychotherapy*, 13, 307–317.

Jakobson, R. (1956). Two Aspects of Language and Two Types of Aphasic Disturbances. In R. Jakobson (Ed.). (1971) *Selected Writings- Word and Language* (Vol. II), Den-Haag- Paris: Mouton, pp. 239–259.

Janet, P. (2010). *Obsessions and Psychasthenia* (trans., Michael W. Adamowicz), LICSW, LLC. [incomplete reference]

Klein, M. (1945). Love, Guilt and Reparation. *International Journal of Psycho-Analysis*, 26, 11–33.

Lacan, J. ([1958] 2007). *Écrits* (trans., Bruce Fink). London: W.W. Norton.

Lacan, J. (1977). The Function and Field of Speech and Language in psychoanalysis. In *Ecrits* (trans., A. Sheridan). New York: Norton, pp. 30–113.

Lacan, J. (1988). *The Seminar of Jacques Lacan. Book I. Freud's Papers on Technique, 1953–54* (trans., John Forrester). New York: Norton; Cambridge: Cambridge University Press.

Lacan, J. (1992). *The Seminar of Jacques Lacan, Book VII: The Ethics of Psychoanalysis* (trans., D. Porter). New York: Norton.

Laplanche, J., & Pontalis, J.-B. (1973). *The Language of Psychoanalysis* (trans., Donald Nicholson-Smith). London: Karnac Books.

Lucas, R. (1992). The Psychotic Personality: A Psychoanalytic Theory and its Application in Clinical Practice. *Psychoanalytic Psychotherapy, 6,* 73–79.

Mallinger, A. (1984), The Obsessive Myth of Control. *Journal of the American Academy for Psychoanalytic Dynamic Psychiatry, 12,* 147–165.

Matte-Blanco, I. (1975). *The Unconscious as Infinite Sets. An Essay in Bi-Logic.* London: Duckworth.

Matte-Blanco, I. (1988). *Thinking, Feeling and Being. Clinical Reflections on the Fundamental Antinomy of Human Beings and the World.* London: Routledge (New Library of Psychoanalysis, Vol 5).

McDougall, J. (1999). *Theatres of the Mind* (trans., Mirjam Kraus). Tel Aviv: Dvir.

Munich, R. (1986). Transitory Symptom Formation in the Analysis of an Obsessional Character. *Psychoanalytic Study of the Child.* New Haven, CT: Yale University Press, Vol. 44, pp. 525–536.

Nagera, H. (1978). *Obsessional Neurosis: Developmental Psychopathology.* New York: Aronson.

O'Connor, J. (2007). The Dynamics of Protection and Exposure in the Development of Obsessive-Compulsive Disorder. *Psychoanalytic Psychology, 24,* 464–474.

Ogden, T. H. (1989). *The Primitive Edge of Experience.* Northvale, NJ: Jason Aronson; London: Karnac Books.

Salzman, L. (1985). *Treatment of the Obsessive Personality.* New York: Aronson.

Segal, H. (1957). Notes on Symbol Formation. *International Journal of Psycho-Analysis, 38,* 391–397.

Steiner, J. (1987). The Interplay between Pathological Organizations and the Paranoid-Schizoid and Depressive Positions. *International Journal of Psycho-Analysis, 68,* 69–80.

Winnicott, D. W. (1965). *The Maturational Process and the Facilitating Environment.* London: The Hogarth Press.

# Chapter 5

# Screen confessions: a fresh analysis of perpetrators' "Newspeak"

The perfect crime, as Jean-François Lyotard (1988) claimed, consists not of killing the victim but rather of obtaining the silence of the witness, the deafness of the judges and the inconsistency of the testimony. If one neutralizes the addressor, the addressee and the significance of the testimony, the result is that there is no referent: no crime has been committed. When, in other words, the witness is blind, the judge is deaf and the testimony has lost coherence and meaning, the crime goes unregistered and hence allegedly never happened.

This chapter focuses on the ways in which the perpetrator erases the referent by silencing her or his "inner witness" (Amir, 2012) and inner judge, turning the entire testimonial text into a false representation of a coherent discourse that in fact undermines its own validity. This erasure, as I will show, is achieved by the emergence of a double language, marked by a dissociation between explicit and implicit meaning: While claiming to generate meaning and adhering to a chronological sequence, this language creates what George Orwell (1949) called "Newspeak": a language that rewrites factual and emotional history alike. This Newspeak yields a phenomenon that I call "screen confessions": voluntary confessional texts produced by perpetrators of their own free will, which share the main characteristic of subtly and unconsciously subverting themselves. The present chapter looks at the linguistic mechanisms by means of which the confessional text transforms itself into a form of subtle camouflage, covering up for another confessional text that either cannot be realized in language or eludes language as it is being realized.

DOI: 10.4324/9781003194071-5

The notion of "screen confessions" was chosen to allude to Freud's 'screen memories (1899). Unlike the notion of screen memory—which refers to the way in which a relatively marginal memory sometimes covers another emotionally charged one that cannot be remembered—the notion of screen confession refers not to memory itself, but to how it is construed in language. Omitted from this kind of confession are not the concrete facts, but their meaning. Distortion or error, thus, do not inhere in the factual details, but in the syntax that interferes in different ways with the original (true) utterance, taking away its meaning even if all of its components are accurate and correct.

This brings to mind Fromm's notion (1941/1994) of the social character. In his discussion of a given culture or society's mediations of what can or cannot penetrate consciousness, Fromm discusses three socially conditioned filters: language, logic and social taboo. In the case of language, Fromm points out that the ability of certain affective experiences to enter consciousness depends on the degree to which a particular language can accommodate the potential experience. The whole structure of language, its grammar, syntax and so on, acts as a kind of template for aspects of experience (Durkin, 2014; Fromm, 1941/1994). Thus, language colludes with cultural and social taboos by means of keeping the culture's unspeakable from being thought and uttered.

Theodor Adorno (1978) writes:

> The leaders are generally oral character types [...]. The famous spell they exercise over their followers seems largely to depend on their orality: language itself, devoid of its rational significance, functions in a magical way and furthers those archaic regressions which reduce individuals into members of crowds. (p. 132)

What is this linguistic magic?

The perpetrator's language serves, in fact, as a "pseudo-language" (Amir, 2014), one which produces "correct" speech that lacks truthfulness. While being perfectly eloquent, it serves as a partition between the individual and her or his inner world, and eventually comes to insulate the person from the truth s/he cannot bear, instead of being the tool by means of which this truth can be expressed.

Pseudo-language is an "attack on linking" (Bion, 1959), aiming to destroy the ability to be conscious of both external and internal reality. One efficient way of achieving this is by the annihilation of any linking that would lead to verbal thought. The link under attack is the one responsible for any fertile connection, whether between mother and baby, analyst and patient, the various parts of the self, or a certain pre-conception and its realization. Once the link has been destroyed, symbolization becomes impossible.

Perpetrators' language manifests many sophisticated forms of this annihilation of linking. These forms will be demonstrated here through the analysis of various World War II testimonial texts, as well as a close reading of Jonathan Littell's The Kindly Ones (2009)—a fictional autobiography describing the life of a former officer in the SS who, decades later, tells the story of a crucial part of his life when he was an active member of the security forces of the Third Reich.

The first thinker to discuss the collective perpetrator's unique use of language was Hannah Arendt (1963), who focused on Eichmann's consistent use of "stock phrases and self-invented clichés" as well as his reliance on "officialese" (*Amtssprache*) and the euphemistic *Sprachregelung*, all aimed at presenting his actions as marginal, on the one hand, and inevitable on the other; as part, that is, of a general mechanism that removes the individual's responsibility for her or his actions. The accomplices in the plan to annihilate the Jews used a neutral verbal mode—"final solution", "mercy death", "euthanasia" and "special treatment"—instead of "extermination". This deployment of language, Arendt argues, played an important part in keeping the general public in the dark. But it also served, and not less importantly, to allow those who participated in the genocide to avoid confronting the clash between their current actions and their former moral norms (p. 86), enabling them in that way not to know their own deeds.

Arendt writes about Eichmann:

> Whether writing his memories in Argentina or in Jerusalem, whether speaking to the police examiner or to the court, what he said was always the same, expressed in the same words. The longer one listened to him, the more obvious it became that his inability to speak was closely connected with an inability to *think*

[...]. No communication was possible with him, not because he lied but because he was surrounded by the most reliable of all safeguards against the words and the presence of others, and hence against reality as such. (p. 44)

Elsewhere, Arendt quotes Eichmann commenting on himself: "Officialese is my only language" (pp. 43–44). Arendt made a brave and subversive effort, in more than one way ahead of its time, to understand this singular pathology of the perpetrator's language. As she listened to this language, she noticed in it various forms of inversion. She described, for instance, the "trick" Himmler used to overcome the "animal compassion" human beings normally experience in the face of physical suffering, including Germans who witnessed their victims' pain:

[...] it consisted in turning these instincts around, as it were, in directing them towards the self. So that instead of saying: What horrible things I did to people!, the murderers would be able to say: What horrible things I had to watch in the pursuance of my duties, how heavily the task weighed upon my shoulders! (p. 93)

This inversion of positions is, indeed, a key syntactic rule of the perpetrator's language. Often in testimonies (for instance, those given to the South African Truth and Reconciliation Commission), perpetrators consider themselves victims of the regime rather than responsible for it. Himmler's solution, however, represents a higher level of sophistication. Here we have a linguistic solution that transforms the one who *causes* the suffering into *the object* of suffering, while dropping the actual object of suffering, i.e., the victim, from the entire syntactic structure. Now the perpetrator—who caused the suffering—occupies both ends of the statement, constituting both subject and object of the act. Where is the victim? In this scene, dominated throughout by the perpetrator, the victim has become reduced to being a mere accessory by means of which the perpetrator causes the suffering which she or he, due to their total commitment to their mission, has to endure.

The victim's elision from the syntactic structure is not accidental. It reflects the subtle and consistent ways by which the perpetrator's language eliminates the meaning of the events it describes. As I will show, however, it is not only the victim whom this language obscures. In the end, through a circular and no less confounding move, it makes the perpetrator him or herself, qua speaking and thinking subject, superfluous. In committing such atrocities, Himmler erases not merely his animal feelings toward his victims' suffering—as Arendt put it—but also his most vital feelings concerning himself. He erases, no more and no less, any relation regarding self and world, splitting, in Waintrater's (2015) words, the living I from the speaking I.

One telltale sign of the perpetrator's language, evident across all types of testimony, whether of collective or of individual perpetrators (Dilmon, 2004, 2007), is the use of the passive grammatical form. The accounts of Nazi officers, for instance, show frequent use of passive rather than active constructions, with many occurrences of "were shot" or "were forced" rather than "I shot" or "I forced". Unsurprisingly, the testimonies of those who refused orders are marked, in contrast, by the use of the first person singular and the active mode. This feature conveys the manner in which perpetrators enlist language to remove the ethical register from their account, i.e., to hide and camouflage their responsibility and the fact that they acted voluntarily, even where they employ this language to reveal the factual truth.

Littell's protagonist, Max Aue puts it this way:

> In correspondence, in speeches too, passive constructions dominated: "it has been decided that …," "the Jews have been conveyed to the special treatment," "this difficult task has been carried out," and so things were done all by themselves, no one ever did anything, no one acted, they were actions without actors, which is always reassuring, and in a way they weren't even actions, since by the special usage that our National Socialist language made of certain nouns, one managed, if not completely to eliminate verbs, at least to reduce them to the state of useless (but nonetheless decorative) appendages, and in that way, you did without even action, there were only facts, brute realities, either already present or waiting for their inevitable accomplishment […]. (pp. 630–632)[1,2]

Aue, however, is saying more than this:

> *Endlösung*: the "Final Solution." But what a beautiful word! It had
> not always been a synonym for extermination, though: since the
> beginning, people had called for, when it came to the Jews, an
> *Endlösung*, or else a *völlige Lösung* (a complete solution) or also an
> *allgemeine Lösung* (a general solution), and according to the period,
> this meant exclusion from public life or exclusion from economic life
> or, finally, emigration. Then, little by little, the signification had slid
> toward the abyss, but without the signifier changing, and it seemed
> almost as if this final meaning had always lived in the heart of the
> word, and that the thing had been attracted, drawn in by it, by its
> weight, its fabulous gravity, into that black hole of the mind, toward
> the point of singularity. [...] Perhaps that, at the bottom, was the
> reason for our *Sprachregelungen*, quite transparent finally in terms
> of camouflage, but useful for keeping those who used these words
> and expressions – special treatment, transported onward, treated
> appropriately, change of domicile, or executive measures – between
> the sharp points of their abstraction. (pp. 630–631)

The perpetrator's language opens an abyss between signifier and
signified. This abyss makes it possible to hygienically articulate unspeakable acts, but over and beyond this linguistic split manifest in
the overt communication, it also facilitates an internal split, within
the speaker, between act and thought. What becomes possible is the
erasure not only of the link between signifier and signified, but also of
the link between the deliverer of the word and the word itself. Thus,
eventually, both the subject upon whom these acts are visited as well
as the subject who perpetrates them (the speaking subject) are annihilated as subjects of and in language.

Aue continues:

> Our system, our state, couldn't care less about the thoughts of its
> servants. It was all the same to the State whether you killed Jews
> because you hated them or because you wanted to advance your
> career or even, in some cases, because you took pleasure in it. It
> did not mind, either, if you did not hate the Jews and the Gypsies

and the Russians you were killing, and if you took absolutely no
pleasure in eliminating them [...]. It did not even mind, in the end,
if you refused to kill them [...]. (p. 131)

The system is not only indifferent to its servants' thoughts: it prefers
they would not think at all. For such a system to stay in place, its
servants must encounter two opposite (dissociated) experiences: The first
is the experience that one is participating in '[...] something crucial, and
that if [one] could understand it then [one would] understand everything
and could finally rest' (p. 131). The second is the experience that no
individual effort of understanding or will matters to one's participation
in the system: it is one's body that is recruited, not one's thought.
   This conflation of grandiosity and total self-effacement, of a sense
of mission that coincides with the total abrogation of the emissary,
creates a vacuum within the subject.

> I'm saying this to you, just to you. The murder of the Jews
> doesn't serve any real purpose. [...] It has no economic or
> political usefulness, it has no finality of a practical order. On
> the contrary, it's a break with the world of economics and
> politics. It's a waste, pure loss. That's all it is. So it can have only
> one meaning: an irrevocable sacrifice, which binds us once and
> for all, prevents us from ever turning back. (p. 142)

Once one takes part in such an act of annihilation, the subject falls
hostage to it. It is now impossible to withdraw, either concretely or
mentally. As a result, the act itself becomes, in a circular way, its own
cause and aim, as the subject who carries it out is simultaneously
being squashed by it. As Aue states, "[a]n SS-Mann should be an
idealist: he cannot do his work and at the same time fornicate with
the prisoners and fill up his pockets" (p. 596).
   Further on he claims:

> But, still, there is a distinction: if a member of the SS has a Jew
> killed in the context of superior orders, that's one thing; but if he
> has a Jew killed to cover his embezzlements, or for his own
> perverted pleasure, as also happens, that's another thing, that's a
> crime. Even if the Jew is to die anyway. (p. 597)

But what, after all, is this distinction? One murder is an act committed in the name of the law, while another comes to conceal the violation of the law. The SS officer is convinced that killing Jews is "in the name of the law", i.e., an act by which she or he fulfills their highest duty. Breaches of the law (rape, theft, and murder in order to cover up acts of rape and theft) then come to be seen as pathological and criminal acts relative to the lawful act of the planned murder. Is there a real difference, though, between these two acts of murder? The internal paradox is so deeply buried in Max Aue's narrative that it is almost impossible to pinpoint. It inheres in the fact that the law, which features as the "suprerior orders" of this narrative, actually undermines any order. Where one is made to assume that mass murder is in the name of the law, the assumption that law or order exists at all crumbles. The text Aue produces here is void of meaning simply because its basic premise is unthinkable; because when the first part of this paragraph ("if a member of the SS has a Jew killed in the context of superior orders, that's one thing") is so groundless, the entire second part ("but if he has a Jew killed to cover his embezzlements, or for his own perverted pleasure, as also happens, that's another thing, that's a crime"), which depends on it, collapses along with it. It is void of meaning because in order for such a sentence to pass, the ears of one's inner judge must be sealed as well as the mouth of one's inner witness. In Lyotard's words, the referent must be erased, or, in those of Bion (1962), the thinking apparatus must be attacked: that of the speaker no less than that of the listener.

Arendt (1963) writes:

> Eichmann, asked by the police examiner if the directive to avoid "unnecessary hardships" was not a bit ironic, in view of the fact that the destination of these people was certain death anyhow, did not even understand the question, so firmly was it still anchored in his mind that the unforgivable sin was not to kill people but to cause unnecessary pain. (p. 96)

Eichmann's stance illustrates another form of attack on linking, manifested in the creation of a false hierarchy of values, one in which the preservation of a low moral value features to conceal the breach of a high moral value. Another illustration of this false hierarchy can be found in a letter by Captain Wolfgang Hoffmann, quoted in its entirety in Daniel Goldhagen (1996): Hoffmann was responsible for the slaughter of tens of thousands of Jews, but protested indignantly against the claim that he or his men could have robbed Poles of food. This ostensibly marginal contradiction, which might easily escape the reader's attention, discloses this perpetrator's way of construing the traumatic reality by camouflaging the a-morality of the massacre by a pseudo-moral vigilance. In this manner, the commandment "Thou shalt not kill" is silenced not by denying the murderous acts themselves but by the vociferous defense of the precept "Thou shalt not steal", which thus comes to serve as a cover up.

> [...] no one had a choice, no one asked anyone's consent, since everyone was interchangeable, victims as well as executioners. For the Russians, as for us, man counted for nothing; the nation, the State were everything; and in this sense we saw our reflection in each other. (Littell, 2009, p. 102)

Freud's group theory (1921) suggests that the fascist demagogue, much like the hypnotist, stirs in the subject the archaic idea of a paramount and dangerous personality toward whom only a passive masochistic attitude is possible, and to whom one's will has to be surrendered. The uncanny and coercive characteristics of group formations may be traced back to their origin in the primal horde: the leader of the group is still the dreaded primal father; the group still longs to be governed by unrestricted force; it has an extreme passion for authority; it has a thirst for obedience. The primal father is the group ideal, and it governs the ego in the place of the ego ideal (Freud, 1921; Adorno, 1951, p. 24). Positing a great other (the leader, the state, the nation) as the exclusive power makes it possible to ignore the life of any private person, whether victim or hangman.

The thesis of the superhuman always involves the erasure of the subhuman and eventually the superhuman too: both are sacrificed in the name of the great other, the latter by dying and the former by becoming executors. The belief that "man counted for nothing; the nation, the State were everything" thus serves two objectives. First, by making the human individual superfluous, it allows the hangman to kill, at one blow, both his fellow human and his own human feelings. Second, it confirms the hypothesis of the hangman as victim, backing up all hangmen's arguments that they, too, were victims of the regime which they chose to obey. In other words, this belief posits the great other as responsible for what we may usefully illustrate with a chess game: it enables those who move the chess pieces to think of themselves as being only one step removed from the pieces they move, and thus to perceive both themselves and their victims as inanimate objects rather than living beings.

Many SS officers after World War II admitted that they have been motivated by a feeling that, if they managed to overcome their "repugnance" toward their own actions, this would make them more faithful soldiers in the service of a greater power for the sake of which they must overcome their human limitations. This is another linguistic circularity: the expression "human limitation", which usually refers to a person's difficulty in restraining her or his hostile feelings and summoning the best of their "humanity", is here transformed into a perception of human-ness itself as a limitation that prevents one, with its "inferior" and "animal-like" emotions such as compassion and remorse, to carry out the required actions against humanity.

When Aue, in the course of an execution, hears his friend humming a song ("The earth is cold, the earth is sweet, dig, little Jew, dig deep"), he is shocked:

> I have known Bohr for some time now, he was a normal man, he had no particular animosity against the Jews, he did his duty as he was told; but obviously, it was eating at him, he wasn't reacting well. (p. 88)

Aue is dismayed when he hears his friend humming because he understands that the latter is becoming identified with his actions. Professionalism, as Aue sees it, and as it is also defined in Bollas' (1992) paper on the fascist state of mind, is the exact opposite of this state of mind: Professionalism, on this view, is the ability to overcome human identifications, to go beyond any feelings of love or hatred, and execute orders hygienically simply because they are orders. "He wasn't reacting well" means that he had regressed to being a human subject, full of hatred in this case. But hate is an aspect of human feelings no less than compassion or love. The perpetrator's language tries to divest itself of any sign of humanity as she or he perceives it: pleasure, hate, compassion, grief. It is driven by the attempt to disconnect, split and undo, not by the wish to create a link (Bion, 1959) between the speaker and her or his actions, or between these actions and the speaker's feelings or values. Disconnection and disavowal, it turns out, is not merely the inevitable outcome of these actions: it is the prerequisite for committing them in the first place.

> Questioned after the war, each one of these people said: What, me, guilty? The nurse didn't kill anyone, she only undressed and calmed the patients, ordinary tasks in her profession. The doctor didn't kill anyone either, he merely confirmed a diagnosis according to criteria established by higher authorities. The worker who opened the gas spigot, the man closest to the actual act of murder in both time and space, was fulfilling a technical function under the supervision of his superiors and doctors. The workers who cleaned out the room were performing a necessary sanitary job [...]. The policeman was following his procedure, which is to record each death and certify that it has taken place without any violation of the laws in force. So who is guilty? [...] why should the worker assigned to the gas chamber be guiltier than the worker assigned to the boilers, the garden, the vehicles? The same goes for every facet of this immense enterprise. (Littell, 2009, p. 19)

An appalling illustration of this type of distancing is Milgram's (1974) (in)famous experiment, which, presenting itself to participants as concerning processes of learning, led the latter to administer increasingly powerful electric shocks to members of the research team, presented as participants who seemed to be giving the wrong answers. Sixty-five percent of the participants administered the maximum—apparently lethal—electric shock. Many participants perspired, stuttered, trembled—indicating that they were not unaware of what they were doing and the possible consequences, yet they did as they were told. The instruction that caused them to push the button was "the experiment requires that you continue". These words, carefully chosen so that they would not describe the task as one subject acting on another subject, framed the setting as one in which an object acts on behalf of the experiment on another object. They masked, at least as far as the true participants (the ones who were encouraged to administer the electric shocks) were concerned, the fact that the situation included two actual subjects. But something else, too, can be observed: the longer the chain of command, and the less significant the role of the person in this chain, the easier it is for this person to deny the overall meaning of the orders she or he obeys. As the chain grows longer, the details of the act it accomplishes grow vaguer, fuzzier and more incomprehensible. When all a person is required to do is push a button during a scientific experiment, she or he will not consider themselves the cause of another person's death, a person who momentarily is also perceived as an object hooked up to the other end of an electric wire rather than a fellow human being, and who—like the one who pushes the button—is nothing but a component in an experiment, an object in the service of something larger: the research, the experiment, science itself.

Littell (2009) writes:

> Undeniably, we were killing a lot of people. That seemed atrocious to me, even if it was inevitable and necessary. But one has to confront atrocity; one must always be ready to look inevitability and necessity in the face and accept the consequences that result from them; closing your eyes is never an answer. (pp. 80–81)

The catch of this formulation is in the syntactic placement of "inevitability and necessity" as a given (constant) rather than a variable. As matters are presented in the above quotation, there is this given called "inevitability and necessity", and the essential question about what we decide to call inevitable and necessary" is replaced by the question of whether we are looking this "inevitability and necessity" in the eye or closing our eyes in front of it. In this manner, the true focus of the sentence shifts to a false focus: The question about the courage to look at the inevitable and necessary masks the question of whether the thing we do or do not look at is really inevitable and necessary.

Another illustration of this shift of focus and the denial it makes possible can be found in the testimony of Albert Fischer, a staff member in Lublin during World War II. In his testimony, Fischer describes another staff member, Max Dietrich, who was known for his extreme cruelty toward the Jewish prisoners. His testimony, quoted in its entirety in Goldhagen (1996), focuses on one incident where Dietrich beat a prisoner until he lost consciousness. Dietrich then forced other prisoners to pour water on his face, and when he woke up, forced him to eat his own feces. At this moment, Fischer states: "I left because it disgusted me". The testimonial text carries here an almost invisible ambiguity: it can be understood as a statement of disagreement with Dietrich's cruel actions; but it can also be received in its simple concreteness: Fischer did not turn away because his friend's cruelty disgusted him, but because the sight of the man eating his own feces made him sick. Thus, the overt declaration of "turning away", allegedly "taking a stand", may mask the possibility that what made him turn away was not his empathy toward the human prisoner, but rather the opposite: his inability to bear this unbelievable horror-show of the prisoner's naked humanity.

> [...] it must have been this that was disturbing the hierarchy, the idea that the men could take pleasure in these actions. Still, everyone who participated in them took some form of pleasure in them – that seemed obvious to me. Some, visibly, enjoyed the act itself, but these could be regarded as sick men, and it was right to ferret them out and give them other tasks, even punish them if they overstepped the bounds. As for the others, whether the actions repelled them or left them indifferent, they carried them out from a sense of duty and obligation, and thus drew pleasure from their devotion, from their ability to carry out such a difficult task despite their disgust and apprehension: "But I take no pleasure in killing", they often said, finding their pleasure, then, in their rigour and their righteousness. (Little, p. 98)

Even-Tzur and Hadar (2017), following Lacan and Žižek, suggest a distinction between the identification of the perpetrator with a

"Living Father" versus the identification of the perpetrator with a "Dead Father":

> The writings of Lacan and his followers delineate the "Living Father" and the "Dead Father" as two opposite "ideal types" of identification figures that provide self-legitimation settings for those who represent the governmental authority and its power: thus, the identification of an agent of Law [...] with a "Living Father" [...] expresses such a belligerent and tyrant subject position that it does not seek any legitimacy or justification of its authority. The father is "living" in a sense similar to the vitality of the tyrant father of the primeval tribe in "Totem and Taboo", who takes pleasure in his power to rule, intimidate and determine arbitrary rules that he is not subjected to personally. On the other hand, the identification of an agent of Law with a "Dead Father" is identification with a fair, equal law that does not represent personal interests and desires. The father is "dead" or "castrated" in the sense that he does not experience absolute *Jouissance* but is, too, restricted by the law (Lacan, 1959/2006, 1960/2006; Žižek, 1994, 1999). (p. 5)

Taking Even-Tzur and Hadar's ideas one step forward, the split between the Living Father and the Dead Father, or between the sadistic parts and the obedient parts, may occur not only between different perpetrators (who may divide into those who identify with the Living Father and take sadistic pleasure in their power, versus those who perceive themselves as merely obedient and take no pleasure from it), but also within the individual perpetrator. One may assume that both modes of identification exist within every perpetrator with varying degrees of dominance. Thus, a perpetrator's confessional text may expose not only his or her dominant mode of identification, but also the relation and interaction between the two modes.

One example of such an interaction may be found in Aue's words when he recounts the story of Leontius in Plato's *Republic*:

> Leontius, the son of Aglaion, coming up one day from the Piraeus, under the north wall on the outside, observed, near the executioner, some dead bodies lying on the ground; and he felt a

desire to look at them, and at the same time loathing the thought he tried to turn away. For a time he struggled with himself, and covered his eyes, till at length, overcome by the desire, he forced his eyes wide open with his fingers, and running up to the bodies, exclaimed, "There! You devils! Gaze your fill at the beautiful spectacle!" (Littell, 2009, p. 98)

Leontius' eyes open not onto the corpses, but onto his own desire to look at them and his prurient, perverse pleasure at the contact with death thus afforded. Touching the dead body, or the dying body, also imparts a transcendence of death, as George Bataille (1957) claims while discussing acts of sacrifice, and as Bollas (1995) points out in his consideration of the psychodynamics of the serial murderer. Contact with death confers a certain immortality on the observer, who becomes able, in an illusory and grandiose manner, to pass through the moment of death itself and remain alive. Thus, Leontius covers his eyes in the name of his identification with the Dead Father, while simultaneously being drawn to look *ad nauseam* in the name of the Living Father who becomes drunk on the power derived from the other's death to confirm his own immortality.

The screening quality of the perpetrator's confession is thus associated with the fact that it has a two-fold function: while the explicit act of confession restores the position of the Dead Father—who is restricted by the law—the implicit act of confession comes to camouflage the Living Father who takes pleasure from his power. While the explicit act aims to constitute the subject as a subject within language, its implicit counterpart erases him or her as one. In order to maintain this complex structure, the perpetrator must at one and the same time confess and subvert this confession through the constitution of a *screen confession*, a compensatory confession. Together these dyads (the Living Father and the Dead Father; the speaker as a subject of language and the speaker as a subject erased by language; language as an act of linking versus language as an attack on linking) make up the language rules used by perpetrators of all kinds. For instance, the use of passive constructions, along with the third person and first person plural, rather than active constructions and the first person singular, not only removes the speaker from the event s/he describes, but also aims to extend the splitting between the "Dead Father" and the "Living Father", thus keeping out of consciousness the pleasure that the use of the first person singular and the active constructions would reveal. The use of "we" distributes pleasure among the many, while the use of the passive helps speakers to place themselves in a masochistic position in order to mask their own sadism.

The common displacement of the victim position from the victim to the victimizer serves the same purpose: as the victimizer shifts attention to the "alleged injustice" of the law, he or she sets aside what Kant and Arendt called "reflexive judgment" (i.e., responsibility for personal injustice and the personal "regime" or "law" that allowed one to act in this particular way). The ambiguity and circularity of the perpetrator's language have a similar goal: taking the guise of logic (expressed in a "given", a "basic assumption" that is repeated and taken for granted) and morality, they allow one to construct a false hierarchy and a psychotic logic.

Piera Aulagnier (2001) argues that "psychotic potentiality" is a condition in which the infant has to fend off the "death wish" the mother directs at him or her from their very birth. This wish is not conscious, but camouflages itself, finding expression in behaviors of a type that often undergo a didactic rationalization. The mother might, for instance, justify harsh and violent behaviors by referring to the need to draw a line or to instill rules of proper conduct. The more intense the mother's death wish, the harder it becomes to repress, and the harder it is to repress—the more destructively it operates within the infant-mother relationship.

Aulagnier argues that the total control the mother exercises over the child's thoughts involves a denial (initially hers, but it becomes the child's as well) of her death wish in relation to him. If he doesn't think what she forbids him to think, he will not know whatever she forbids him to know. Aulagnier uses Orwell's *1984* to illustrate how, in the Newspeak of the psychotic's mother, everything that might have created a true contact between the child's emotional experience and the maternal wish as a factor in that experience is removed. The child does not have the right to understand what she or he perceives. This prohibition on understanding may in time transform into a prohibition on memory and lead to the erasure of entire parts of the child's historical narrative (Aulagnier, 2001; Amir, 2014). The mother of the future psychotic, similar to the collective and the individual perpetrator, creates an environment in which language, rather than forging a link between a person and her or his experience, severs between them. This dissociation is typical of both victim and perpetrator.

In his chapter "The Fascist State of Mind", Bollas (1992) argues that, in this mindset, the space previously taken up in the symbolic order by a plurality of meanings is now colonized by slogans. As long as the internal regime was democratic, words and symbols were free to associate with other words and symbols. But when representation becomes obstructed, signifiers lose this freedom. The elimination of the symbolic and the plural is the fascist regime's first act of murder: this is because the symbolic, always unbinding any fixed meaning and undermining any act of homogenization, is the true subversive element of thought.

Arendt (1963) observes similar qualities in Eichmann's language: "He was genuinely incapable of uttering a single sentence that was not a cliché" (p. 44). Here we must remember that a cliché is not merely a turn to the lowest common denominator, as is commonly assumed, but also comes to economize on the act of thinking and make it superfluous: it fixates thought itself as a field of manacled, saturated meanings (Bion, 1962). "Language can function as a 'living' system of signs which grants meaning to the encounter between the internal world and reality', writes Roth (2017)," and it can also serve as a 'fossil' in and of itself—a 'dead' sign system, which 'points toward' but never establishes a 'link with' what is signified. In this case, the sign functions without its symbolic quality" (p. 186).

Screen confessions are not only linguistic fossils, as Roth argues, but also take on a radioactive quality, as Gampel (1999, 2017) has put it. As such they have an impact that goes beyond the immediate to the intergenerational; they influence, over and beyond their intended recipients, those who are their passive audience and who unwittingly absorb the radiation.

By dismantling the language in which she or he thinks their actions, the perpetrator excludes not only the victims from the story but him or herself as well. As long as the perpetrator remains outside the story, her or his testimonial text constitutes an "empty event" or an "event without witness" (Felman and Laub, 1992): an event from which the perpetrator, the alleged most reliable witness of her or his own actions, is absent. Caruth (1996), dealing with post-traumatic phenomena, writes about the "traumatic paradox" in which the most direct contact with the violent event may take place through the very inability to know it (pp. 91–92). Trauma is not only an experience, she claims, but also the failure to experience: not the threat itself, but the fact that the threat was recognized as such only a moment too late. Since it was not experienced "in time", the event is fated from now on not to be fully known (p. 62). However, not only the victims are doomed to not know what happened to them. Perpetrators, too, suffer from a similar traumatic miss.

When the disease is the splitting of language, the one possible basis for recovery is to reclaim language. Such reclaiming, in the case of perpetrators' confessions, implies reintroducing the linking function. This means restoring coherence between the explicit and implicit contents, between words and emotional experience, and perhaps more than anything, it implies the rehabilitation of the referent, i.e., the reclaiming of the function of the inner witness, the function of the inner judge and the function of creating meaning so that the testimonial event will turn from a pseudo-performance into a vital event—one in which the subject, facing her or his concrete or imaginary victims, will be fully present.

## Notes

1 From The Kindly Ones by Jonathan Littell: Copyright (c) 2009 by Jonathan Littell. Englishlanguage translation copyright (c) 2009 by Charlotte Mandell. Used by permission of HarperCollins Publishers.
2 From *The Kindly Ones* by Jonathan Littell published by Vintage. Copyright © Jonathan Littell 2006. Reprinted by permission of The Random House Group Limited.

## References

Adorno, T. (1978). Freudian Theory and the Pattern of Fascist Propaganda. In A. Arato and E. Gebhardt (Eds.). *The Essential Frankfurt School Reader*. Oxford: Blackwell, Part 1: pp. 118–137.

Amir, D. (2012). The Inner Witness. *International Journal of Psycho-Analysis*, *93*(4), 879–896.

Amir, D. (2014). *Cleft Tongue: The Language of Psychic Structures*. London: Karnac Books.

Arendt, H. (1963). *A Report on the Banality of Evil*. New York: The Viking Press.

Aulagnier, P. (2001). *The Violence of Interpretation* (trans., A. Sheridan). London: Routledge.

Bataille, G. (1957). *Eroticism: Death and Sensuality* (trans., M. Dalwood). San Francisco: City Lights, p. 1986.

Bion, W. R. (1959). Attacks on Linking. *International Journal of Psycho-Analysis*, *40*, 308–315.

Bion, W. R. (1962). A Theory of Thinking. *Second Thoughts*. London and New York: Karnac, Vol. 1984, pp. 110–119.

Bollas, C. (1992). The Fascist State of Mind. *Being a Character: Psychoanalysis and Self Experience*. New York: Routledge, pp. 193–217.

Bollas, C. (1995). The Structure of Evil. *Cracking Up: The Work of Unconscious Experience*. London and New York: Routledge, pp. 180–220.

Caruth, C. (1996). *Unclaimed Experience: Trauma Narrative and History*. Baltimore, MD: Johns Hopkins University Press.

Dilmon, R. (2004). Linguistic Differences Between Lie and Truth in Spoken Hebrew. PhD thesis. Ramat Gan, Israel: Bar-Ilan University.

Dilmon, R. (2007) Fiction or Fact? Comparing True and Untrue Anecdotes. *Hebrew Linguistics*, *59*, 23–42.

Durkin, K. (2014). *The Radical Humanism of Erich Fromm*. New York: Palgrave Macmillan.

Even-Tzur, E. and Hadar, U. (2017). Agents of the Father's Law in a Society of Brothers: A Philosophic and Psychoanalytic Perspective on Legitimate Use of Violence. *International Journal of Law and Psychiatry*, *51* (March–April): 22–32.

Felman, S. and Laub, D. (1992). *Testimony: Crises of Witnessing in Literature, Psychoanalysis, and History*. New York and London: Routledge.

Freud, S. (1899). Screen Memories. *Standard Edition* 3 (1962). London: Hogarth Press, pp. 299–322.

Freud, S. (1921). Group Psychology and the Analysis of the Ego. *Standard Edition* 18 (1955). London: Hogarth Press, pp. 65–144.

Freud, S. (1921/1955). Group Psychology and the Analysis of the Ego. *Standard Edition* 18. London: Hogarth Press, pp. 65–144.

Fromm, E. (1941/1994). *Escape From Freedom*. Henry Holt and Company, New York: Owl Books Edition.

Gampel, Y. (1999). Between the Background of Safety and the Background of Uncanny in the Context of Social Violence. In E. Bott Spillius (Ed. in chief). *Psychoanalysis on the Move*. London: Routledge, pp. 59–74.

Gampel, Y. (2017) Evil. In R. Lazar (Ed.). *Talking about Evil*. London and New York: Routledge, pp. 1–16.

Goldhagen, D. (1996). *Hitler's Willing Executioners: Ordinary Germans and the Holocaust*. New York: Random House.

Lacan, J. (1959/2006). On a Question Prior to any Possible Treatment of Psychosis. *Écrits: The First Complete Edition in English* (trans., B. Fink). New York: W.W. Norton, pp. 445–488.

Lacan, J. (1960/2006). The Subversion of the Subject and the Dialectic of Desire in the Freudian Unconscious. *Écrits: The First Complete Edition in English* (trans., B. Fink). New York: W.W. Norton.

Littell, J. (2009). *The Kindly Ones* (trans., C. Mandell). New York: HarperCollins books.

Lyotard, J.-F. (1988). *The Differend: Phrases in Dispute* (trans., G. Van Den Abbeele). Manchester: Manchester University Press.

Milgram, S. (1974) *Obedience to Authority: An Experimental View*. New York, NY: Harper and Row.

Orwell., G. (1949). *1984*. London: Secker and Warburg.

Roth, M. (2017). The Restorative Power of Reading Literature: From Evil to Dialectics. In R. Lazar (Ed.). *Talking about Evil*. London and New York: Routledge, pp. 181–199.

Waintrater, R. (2015). Body Image and Identity in Victims of Extreme Violence. In E. Sukhanova and H.-O. Tomashoff (Eds.). *Body Image and Identity in Contemporary Society: Psychoanalytic, Social, Cultural and Aesthetic Perspectives*. London and New York: Routledge, pp. 49–55.

Žižek, S. (1994). *The Metastases of Enjoyment: Six Essays on Women and Causality*. London and New York: Verso.

Žižek, S. (1999). *The Ticklish Subject: The Absent Centre of Political Ontology*. London and New York: Verso.

# Chapter 6

# Epilogue

## "Studium" and "Punctum" in psychoanalytic writing: reading case studies through Roland Barthes

The various chapters of Roland Barthes' *Camera Lucida* (1982) accompany him as if he were leafing through his personal photo album. But rather than considering the nostalgic or aesthetic context, this book is a reflection on gaze itself.

How does a reflection on photography line up with thoughts about psychoanalytic writing?

The case study, like the photograph, seeks to take hold of something nearly intangible. It attempts to capture in time, space and language, something whose dynamic presence is elusive. In fact, the very attempt at capturing this object often strips it from its essence. Case studies may be thoroughly accurate on the face of it, while at the same time giving us the uncomfortable sense that they have "deadened" their object in the process.

What is it that escapes the picture which the psychoanalytic writing aims to take? According to Barthes, the Photograph represents that very subtle moment when one is neither subject nor object but a subject who feels he is becoming an object, thus experiencing a micro-version of death. The photographer, Barthes claims, knows this very well, and himself fears this death. It is as if he must exert himself to the utmost to keep the photograph from becoming death (Barthes, 1982, p. 14).

Like the object of the photograph, the object of the psychoanalytic case study shifts as a result of the act of documentation: from being a subject it becomes an object, and therefore runs the risk of being annihilated in the very process of being written up. What makes the case study into an even more complex genre is that its object is the therapeutic act, e.g., a vivid dynamic process rather than a well-defined

DOI: 10.4324/9781003194071-6

figure. Often, all too often, readers find themselves witnessing the ghost of the therapeutic session rather than having a sense of the living event, or, alternatively, come upon a plethora of collected mummifications of the therapeutic act that are the result of the misguided attempt to capture its essence.

Georges Perec struggles with a similar problem in his book *W, or the Memory of Childhood* (1975). The only way for him to preserve the living memory of his childhood is by fragmenting its literary images. Like Barthes, he realizes that the true experience is not what the image actually captures but rather what manages to escape from it. Describing his recollected images, Perec illustrates how the actuality of a picture, rather than residing in the formal facts, inheres in something else that eludes them and yet is made possible by them. Psychoanalytic writing, too, pursues this elusive element when it sets the formal facts or the chronological therapeutic sequence before the lens of its camera. It is when our gaze directs itself at the very center of the picture, that something else, situated in its margins, may enter our field of vision. The only way, however, one can direct one's attention at this is by a non-focused observation. This is the paradox of the case study. In its attempt to capture its object it must puncture the image it aims to present. In order to breathe life into its subject matter, it must perforate the narrative. In Barthes' words—"in order to see a photograph well, it is best to look away or close our eyes" (Barthes, 1982, p. 53).

In this paradoxical process of looking at a photograph, the following two elements come into play: the first is what Barthes calls the *studium*. This is our cultural domain, the vantage point from which we observe the photograph as such. Here reside the assembled types of familiar knowledge by means of which the stimulus we perceive communicates itself to us, entering a recognizable context. The function of the second element, which Barthes calls the *punctum*,[1] is to puncture or disturb the *studium*. The *punctum* reaches through the *studium*'s recognizable co-ordinates, impinging on the observing mind. It is the accident that strikes the gaze. While the *studium* produces an effect of *liking*, not *loving* (thus entertains harmonious relations, whether positive or negative, always within the confines of the intelligible and communicable, with what the photographer meant to convey)—experience in the order of desire comes into play only where there is a *punctum*. Most photographs, says Barthes, provoke only a general and *polite* interest. They have no *punctum* in them. They please or displease the observer without pricking him. They are invested with no more than *studium*, mobilizing a half desire, a "demi-volition". To recognize the *studium* is to encounter the photographer's intentions, i.e., to understand them. The *studium* is a kind of "education" which allows the observer to experience that which establish the photographer's practices, but to experience them "in reverse", investing them with a sort of pleasure, never with delight or pain (Ibid, pp. 27–28).

The *studium* produces the "reverse gear" of the event. The *punctum*, by contrast, is the here and now, the instantaneous. It is the "this is". It shatters the existing categories and regular order of things by making a "hole" or a "wound" in the observer, removing him or her from the *studium*'s common ground to an alien and exposed region within. Once there is a *punctum*, a blind field is created, as if the image launched desire beyond what it permits us to see (Ibid, pp. 57–59).

Something like this happens in Georges Perec's description of a photograph in which he appears at his mother's side in a Parisian park (1975 [2010], p. 49). He renders in minute detail his and her attire, her facial features as well as his own face. On the edge of the photo one may glimpse something that could be part of the overcoat of the person taking the picture, who might be his father; and in the background appears a little girl in a light-colored coat. These two marginal details shed light on the portrait to which this picture is dedicated, the portrait of the absent, which the picture cannot contain: a father who was brutally killed; a younger sister who died soon after her birth. This is an illustration of what Barthes calls the "blind field". The photograph takes on meaning not as a result of the formal details it explicitly presents—and which correspond with the spectator's *studium*—but rather as a result of the marginal details that perforate the frontal image. Thus, it is the blind field, what remains subtly beyond, that achieves the powerful effect of recollection and therefore consists the crux of both the photograph and the photographic experience.

In the genre of the psychoanalytic case study, too, a sharp, unique effect is often created by what is left out of the story or in its margins, unintended, rather than what we well know. These are the zones that lie beyond what's there for all to see, and by means of which we arouse curiosity, desire and the pleasure of seeking. The effect of penetration, of shock, is never achieved by a mass of details and explanations that saturate and satisfy the reader's mind, but by something that whets the appetite, stimulates thought, urging the reader to hold back, as Barthes puts it, instead of activating the usual, passive receptors in front of the textual stimulus. These are the moments when the text gives itself rather than shows itself to us. Only then, we give ourselves to it in return.

In terms of the psychoanalytic case study, then, the *studium* retrospectively reconstructs the therapeutic move. This refers not quite simply to the therapeutic process but also to our use of the psychoanalytic discourse in which we are grounded in order to interpret this process. Here we refer to currently relevant theories in order to validate our understandings and actions, presenting them in this way to both ourselves and our readers in the form of a linear, coherent sequence. The *punctum*, by contrast, is the manner in which the case perforates one's thinking about it. Here linearity collapses, and an unruly element slips into the structured scene which rejects the syntax we have imposed on it and requires new, fresh thinking. A beautiful illustration of the moment the case itself perforates the author's *studium*, is found in a vignette Ronald Britton includes in his *Belief and Imagination* (1998):

The patient opened the mentioned session by saying—"When I came in I thought you looked fed up, not interested, hostile or cold" (Britton, 1998, p. 90). Then he paused briefly, and as if beginning again, said:

It is very interesting, I used the toilet here for the first time. On my way here I felt I had to have a shit, but didn't want to be late so I didn't stop. But I didn't want to do it here. Anyway I came in slightly early to do so. When I was in the car I thought "I have to" and I had a pain. I thought of a condition I was told I had years ago – don't know if you know it – proctalgia fugax, fleeting pain in the anus. (Ibid, pp. 90–91)

Britton writes:

By this time the patient had warmed to the subject, and talked of himself and his experiences in a steadily more expansive way. Clearly, he was now talking to someone he thought of as interested and friendly. However, the sense of something sudden, violent and sinister […], remained in my mind as a disturbing image, but one that had vanished from his discourse, which was easy and relaxed. (Ibid, p. 91)

At this point Britton tells the patient: "You cannot direct your feelings toward me fully, and I think you dare not take your fleeting picture seriously, of me as hostile; so you have covered the picture with words" (Ibid).

The conversation continues in more or less this spirit, and then the patient says:

> I thought last week when I spoke to you about my colleague's anal fissure and you said that it was an example of a condition that gets worse before it gets better [Britton linked it with analysis – DA]... I understood what you meant about dilatation as treatment but I thought you said it with [searching for a word] relish. I thought it showed your...um...can't think of the word... (Ibid, p. 92)

Britton suggests the word is "sadism" and the patient confirms: "that's right, I thought you were sadistic" (Ibid).

What is interesting about this case is that it constitutes a second reading. Britton already used it in another article, in 1995, where it served to show how the patient understood, by the end of the session, that he "seriously entertained a persecutory belief that the analyst might be a dangerous, cruel figure, and that he had been attempting to evade this belief" (Ibid). Britton now offers the same case in order to show that the opposite is true: the interpretations he gave acted to refute the wild notion regarding the analyst's sadism rather than to help the patient to be in touch with it. The interpretation—and the joint reflection following it—came to restore the relations between analyst and patient to their status quo, and to silence the intolerable thought concerning the analyst's sadism. "If he could talk reasonably about these things it meant they need not been taken seriously any longer", Britton writes (Ibid). And so "he thought about himself in order to avoid being himself" (Ibid, p. 93). Britton further writes:

> In this process a belief is not reality tested and finally relinquished, but temporarily overcome by the reassurance of the analytic situation itself. [...] Like the eruption of a child's belief in monsters in the middle of the night, it is overcome by the reassuring presence of the parent for that night, but this lasts only until the next time. Some incarnation of the deadened monster threatens to appear in

the person of the analyst, but the process of the analysis itself becomes the means of banishing it. The analysis retains its *heimlich* (homely) qualities and the individual remains vulnerable to the intrusions of the *unheimlich*, the horrifying known-unknown or unknown-known. (ibid)

I would like to go back at this point to the *punctum* of this case study and to what eventually led, I believe, to the opposite understanding of the same sequence of events. This is the moment when the patient says: "I thought 'I have to' and I had a pain". Since the anus is a type of mouth, it is, like the actual mouth, at risk of expelling what cannot be borne. The patient is locked into his pain because he can neither keep "the thing" inside nor release it. The thing that cannot be released is his discovery of the analyst's pleasure when talking about "dilatation", namely about the dilatation of the patient's anus as an analogy to the analytic act. The patient senses that the analyst enjoys the metaphor, or the idea, or maybe even the act of dilatation itself. He says to him—"I thought it showed your...um...", almost as though he was telling him—"I was suddenly looking at your erect penis". Here Britton hastens to offer the patient the word "sadism" by way of re-placing the "um". But his suggestion, ostensibly a bold interpretation, turns out to be a trap: it transforms sadism from being something vital and terrifying, into something that can be discussed and thereby dis-missed. The psychoanalytic process now undermines both itself and the possibility of true contact. Calling things by their name comes, in fact, to be a way to avoid contact with their insufferable essence.

Taking a look at both of Britton's interpretations of the same ana-lytic moment, one may say that the first—the one that sees calling sadism by its name as an analytic achievement—fits with Barthes' de-scription of the *studium*. It follows the obvious route where the psy-choanalytic process is defined as helping the patient to connect to what has hitherto been out of his or her conscious reach. The second inter-pretation is the *punctum*. This is when the predictable analytic picture is perforated and turns upside down. What seemed to be directed upward now stands revealed as dragging the analysis steeply down into a chasm; what is usually considered to be "doing the job" turns out to actually undo that job. The moment in which the analyst offers the word "sadism" to the patient who seemingly doesn't manage to find it himself, now, in this new interpretation, is revealed as the moment in which he defuses his own sadism. He offers the patient the word to reassure him that there is nothing to be frightened of, as if telling him that when someone calls something by its name—this calling by name takes away its power. But the patient knows better: he knows that "um...", or "your...um..."—pointing to the Real rather than being situated in the symbolic—is more appropriate to what is happening between him and the analyst than the proper word "sadism". He also knows that no sooner than the word captures the thing, the thing, the "um", will vanish. This is why he hesitates, stammers, holds back, a bit like how he tries to avoid visiting the analyst's toilet before the session. It's not just because of the smell it would spread. It's the fear of the analyst's "flushing" the smell down. And so one can say that Britton's interpretation of this case shifts from *studium* to *punctum* when he understands that analysis itself is in danger of turning into an act of "flushing" that comes to restore analytic hygiene and order at the cost of the very thing it is intended to address.

Barthes also notes what Britton pinpoints here, saying that the incapacity to name is a good symptom of disturbance (*Punctum*). The effect is certain but unlocatable, it does not find its sign, it cries out in silence (Barthes, 1982, pp. 51–53). The *punctum* is the Archimedean point (*punctum Archimedis*) from which psychoanalytic writing pulls itself out of the swamp it itself produces. It is an act of reversal.

One wonderful description of how this reversal happens appears in a chapter of Barthes' book entitled "Winter Garden Photograph" (p. 67). Throughout this chapter he tries in vain to find among his family photographs one that reflects his recently deceased, beloved mother: but what he finds, it turns out, are only parts: certain features of her face, a typical gesture, the shape of a hand. What isn't restored to him in those photographs is her *being*. In so far as they are partially true, they are wholly false. The encounter with them consigns him to the terrible *almost* of love, but also with dream's disappointing status—which is why he hates dreams. For he often dreams *about her*, but never dreams *her* (Ibid, pp. 65–66).

Rejecting her later photographs one after another, he finally spots one from her childhood. What he finds there—something distinct in her face, an innocence of posture—conveys the impossible paradox which she retained throughout her life, an "assertion of a gentleness".

For once, photography gave him a sentiment as certain as remembrance. This Winter Garden photograph was for him like the last music Schumann wrote before collapsing, he writes, that first *Gesänge der Frühe* which accords with both his mother's being and his grief at her death.[2] While those "ordinary" photographs were merely analogical, provoking only her identity, not her truth—the Winter Garden photograph was indeed essential, it achieved for him, utopically, "the impossible science of the unique being" (Ibid, pp. 69–70).

Later in the same chapter Barthes writes that what he has lost is not the indispensable, but the irreplaceable (ibid, p. 75). This is exactly what is often missing from the psychoanalytic case study as well. It tries to capture the irreplaceable and yet clings to the indispensable: the tiniest details, the chronological sequence, the attempt to bring the facts together under headings, concepts or theoretical domains. What often goes lost in the process of illustration or generalization is the singular being, the irreducible essence, that radiant core of "The Mother" which Barthes calls "my mother" (Ibid).

It is not a question of accuracy but of reality, Barthes further argues (ibid, p. 80). Likewise, the case study derives its force from the realness and truthfulness it conveys. The most factually exact description, in this sense, is not necessarily more truthful than a masked description which contains invented details. As long as the invention captures this realness and truthfulness it does not offend against the truth. This truthful core does not always have to do with the missing "detail" which creates, as said earlier, a blind spot. Sometimes it is a syntactic mode or a certain rhythm of writing that captures this irreducible, ungeneralizable and singular quality whose necessity turns out to be the necessity of the text itself. This "new *punctum*", as Barthes calls it, which is no longer of form but of intensity, is Time. In front of the photograph of his mother as a child, he tells himself: "she is going to die". He shudders, like Winnicott's psychotic patient, "over a catastrophe which has already occurred" (Ibid, pp. 94–96).

The photograph's intensity, therefore, inheres in the fact that although it seizes a calamity that happened some time ago, it strikes the awed viewer with a sense as though the calamity is about to happen now. The case study, too, includes the inevitable calamity of the analytic process as something that "is bound to occur" rather than as something that belongs to the past. This is the reason why case studies are often written in present tense. Like photographs they exist in a double time zone: past and future merge so that these texts include both the facticity of what has taken place and the tremor of what is going to be (Ibid, pp. 116–117).

Every case study is a work of mourning. It holds on to the object but at the same time seeks to let go of it in order to recreate it in terms of its essence, or of its truth. The details it includes resemble dream contents: they must be remembered in order to be forgotten, written in order to be erased. One could consider the entire process of writing a case study as a journey from the "analogical photographs" to the "Winter Garden photograph": from the possibility to "dream about her" to the possibility of "dreaming her".

The "Winter Garden photograph" is different from the analogical photographs because of what Barthes calls "the air": a kind of intractable supplement of identity, what is given as an act of grace, stripped of any importance; what accomplishes reality—"*that-has-been*"—with truth "*there-she-is!*" (Ibid, p. 113).

At the rare moments when a case study achieves this combination of reality and truth, it takes hold of something not merely in terms of its subject matter but also in terms of its form. I found such a moment in a case description by Michael Eigen, included in his book *Psychic Deadness* (1996):

> She [the patient] used the word "simple" repeatedly: "What I need is simple. It's simply what you'd give a child of your own. The simplest thing in the world".

Eigen continues:

> I feel that simple thing at the center of my being. It shows in my eyes, my tone, my skin. I live from and through it. It is my home. Yet some people see it, and some do not. [...] Where is that simple thread leading to and coming from the heart's center? Where is it when it is lost? How can something I feel so deeply and thoroughly not show? With Janice I felt like a stroke victim who could feel his shining essence unable to break through layers of imprisonment. [...] No uncertainty of locale could be tolerated, and there was no

time. Either I was the one who could do it or not, and I had to be the one to say so.

(Eigen, 1996, pp. 216–217)

"Love me like your own child" (ibid, p. 221), Janice asks him again and again.

Eigen writes:

God, how I love my children! How I can hate them too! Their life kills me off. I come back. I want to kill them and *fight* for my life. [...] How can they escape my wounds, or I theirs? We each have our inner drummers. We are driven to come through – to live. I look at them and feel my death. I look at them and thrill to life. (Ibid, pp. 221–222)

The "air" that this case study captures is not Janice's but that of the very special failure of analysis in the face of her singularity. This failure does not touch us necessarily in terms of its subject-matter—even though it is full of subject matter; it does not reach for generalization even though it allows us to learn about this type of failure a great deal beyond the specific conditions of its occurrence. It is rather written as a lament: a lament about both the pretentiousness and helplessness of psychoanalysis. One could say that Eigen perforates the psycho-analytic world view by means of the intensive and unique encounter he creates between the writing ear and the reading ear, enacting by means of the text's music what this text seeks to bear witness to.

"As a *Spectator* I was interested in Photography only for 'senti-mental' reasons; I wanted to explore it not as a question [...] but as a wound", Barthes writes at the outset of his book (1982, p. 21). The "other (new) *punctum*" he mentions is exactly what pierces the case study when writing explores it not as a question but as a wound. No matter how astute and complex, delving into a case as a question is likely to lead one to a new understanding, not to a new truth. What will be expanded is the person's "knowing about"—not his or her "essential knowing" (Meltzer & Harris-Williams, 1988). Exploring it as a wound, by contrast, brings into play a different quality of linking. These are the rare moments in which the "case study" turns into a "case story": as such, it does not "seize" an understanding or an idea that the readers may find useful, but simply grabs them by the throat.

## Notes

1 The Latin word (*"Punctum"*) designates a wound, a prick, a mark made by a pointed instrument. *Punctum* is also sting, speck, cut, a little hole and a cast of the dice (Ibid, pp. 26–27).
2 This reminds me of Ogden's beautiful essay on mourning:

> Mourning is not simply a form of psychological work; it is a process centrally involving the experience of *making* something, creating something adequate to the experience of loss. What is 'made', and the experience of making it—which together might be thought of as 'the art of mourning'—represent the individual's effort to meet, to be equal to, to do justice to, the fullness and complexity of his or her relationship to what has been lost, and to the experience of loss itself. The creativity involved in the art of mourning need not be the highly developed creativity of the talented artist. The notion of creativity, as I conceive it here, applies equally to 'ordinary creativity', that is, to the creativity of everyday life. What one 'makes' in the process of mourning—whether it be a thought, a feeling, a gesture, a perception, a poem, a response to a poem, or a conversation—is far less important than the experience of making it. (Ogden, 2001, pp. 117–118)

## References

Barthes, R. (1982). *Camera Lucida* (trans., Richard Howard). London: Vintage Publishing.

Britton, R. (1998). *Belief and Imagination*. London: Routledge, in Association With the Institute of Psycho-Analysis.

Britton, R. (1998). Complacency in Analysis and Everyday Life. *In Belief and Imagination*. London: Routledge, in association with the Institute of Psychoanalysis, pp. 82–96.

Eigen, M. (1996). Boa and Flowers. *Psychic Deadness*. London: Jason Aronson, pp. 213–224.

Meltzer, D., & Harris-Williams, M. (1988). Holding the Dream. *The Apprehension of Beauty*. Scotland: Clunie Press, pp. 178–199.

Ogden, T. (2001). Borges and the Art of Mourning. *Conversations at the Frontier of Dreaming*. Northvale, NJ: Jason Aronson/London, pp. 115–152.

Perec, G. (2010). *W or The Memory of Childhood* (trans., D. Bellos). Boston, MA: D.R. Godine (Originally published in 1975).

# Index